AT THE INTERFACE OF
CULTURE AND MEDICINE

AT THE INTERFACE
OF CULTURE
AND MEDICINE

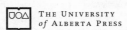

Edited by

Earle H. Waugh

Olga Szafran

Rodney A. Crutcher

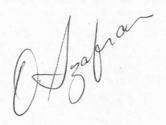

THE UNIVERSITY
of ALBERTA PRESS

Published by

The University of Alberta Press
Ring House 2
Edmonton, Alberta, Canada   T6G 2E1

Copyright © 2011 The University of Alberta Press

Library and Archives Canada Cataloguing in Publication

At the interface of culture and medicine / edited by Earle H. Waugh,
Olga Szafran and Rodney A. Crutcher.

Includes bibliographical references and index.
ISBN 978-0-88864-532-6

1. Medical anthropology. 2. Social medicine. I. Waugh, Earle H.,
1936- II. Szafran, Olga, 1957- III. Crutcher, Rodney A., 1950-

GN296.A8 2011   306.4'61   C2010-908136-6

All rights reserved.
First edition, first printing, 2011.
Printed and bound in Canada by Houghton Boston Printers, Saskatoon, Saskatchewan.
Copyediting by Lisa LaFramboise.
Proofreading by April Hickmore.
Indexing by Adrian Mather.

No part of this publication may be produced, stored in a retrieval system, or
transmitted in any forms or by any means, electronic, mechanical, photocopying,
recording, or otherwise, without the prior written consent of the copyright owner or
a licence from The Canadian Copyright Licensing Agency (Access Copyright). For an
Access Copyright licence, visit www.accesscopyright.ca or call toll free: 1-800-893-5777.

The University of Alberta Press is committed to protecting our natural environment.
As part of our efforts, this book is printed on Enviro Paper: it contains 100% post-
consumer recycled fibres and is acid- and chlorine-free.

The University of Alberta Press gratefully acknowledges the support received for its
publishing program from The Canada Council for the Arts. The University of Alberta
Press also gratefully acknowledges the financial support of the Government of Canada
through the Book Publishing Industry Development Program (BPIDP) and from the
Alberta Foundation for the Arts for its publishing activities.

  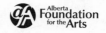

CONTENTS

PREFACE

THE GROWTH OF THE BIOMEDICAL MODEL of health care seems like such a given in Canadian culture that it is difficult to admit that it is one of several embraced around the world. The popularity of the model among so-called advanced societies and its recent enlistment of evidence-based therapies mean that it has come to dominate the field. If we pause to reflect for a moment, we can clearly see that the biomedical model also has a history and that it has evolved along with Western scientific advancement: biomedical knowledge cannot be separate from the culture that promoted it. This removes some of the absolutes often associated with biomedical statements.

The mandate of the Centre for the Cross-Cultural Study of Health and Healing in the Department of Family Medicine, University of Alberta, is to explore the way different cultures have developed and applied medical knowledge. It seemed only natural, then, that the centre should team up with physicians, educators, and practitioners to try to bring clarity to the rather complicated relationship that biomedicine has with other systems of medical knowledge. This book contextualizes this relationship within the contemporary Canadian scene. Canada has developed a rather sophisticated medical system that has some unique elements and is in the process of rapidly diversifying its cultural character through significant immigration from around the world. The result will likely be demands for other systems of health care. It will be helpful for students of health care around the world to know just how Canada is responding to these pressures.

Very early in our collaboration, the editors met together to probe how we could further a discussion within Canada of the way in which medicine relates to culture. In the face of rising ethnic expectations and the flourishing of complementary and alternative therapies, we decided to situate our discussion within the local academy, with the view to drawing on as diverse an approach as possible. While there are limitations to what one book can do, we urged our colleagues to focus attention as much as possible on their recent research, which would bring fresh stances to bear on the interface of culture and medicine. We also hoped to spur additional research on this important topic.

We trust this book will promote a serious engagement between health care professionals and cultural brokers in Canada, and we urge policy development to accommodate the new realities on the ground in this country.

ACKNOWLEDGEMENTS

THIS COLLECTION WOULD NOT HAVE BEEN POSSIBLE without the vigorous support of our academic community. Both the University of Calgary and the University of Alberta provided a fertile ground within which to work. They applauded our probing of the issues in real ways—with financial, institutional, and personal support. We are most grateful to them. Many of the studies have received assistance from various funding agencies, to which we are all indebted.

We especially want to express appreciation to Dr. G. Richard Spooner, Chair of the Department of Family Medicine, University of Alberta, who not only supported the initial idea, but also provided departmental support for the publication of this collection. Funding support was also obtained from the Dr. Scott H. McLeod Family Medicine Memorial Fund and from the University of Calgary. Many of us have had assistance from colleagues in both Edmonton and Calgary, and we want to acknowledge that their input has been seminal for many of our conceptions. We are deeply grateful to Peggy Lewis and Shufen Edmondstone for secretarial assistance with the manuscript. Finally, we appreciate the comments from reviewers and associates of the University of Alberta Press; they have made this a better contribution with their cogent editing and constructive criticism.

Earle H. Waugh
University of Alberta

Olga Szafran
University of Alberta

Rodney A. Crutcher
University of Calgary

INTRODUCTION

Earle H. Waugh

Olga Szafran

Rodney A. Crutcher

MULTICULTURALISM IS A DISTINCTIVE FEATURE of Canadian society. Immigration has shaped the racial, ethnic, and cultural diversity of Canada's population. According to the 2006 census, 18.9% of Canadians and 15.6% of Albertans were born outside of Canada (Statistics Canada, 2007a). More notable, however, is the non-English mother tongue of 42.8% of Canadians (Quebec accounts for half) and 20.9% of Albertans. Since 1971, Canada's policy of "Multiculturalism within a Bilingual Framework" has embraced diversity as a legitimate part of Canadian identity. In 1999, Prime Minister Jean Chrétien stated that "We have established a distinct Canadian way. A Canadian model. A multicultural society populated by people from almost every country in the world. Accommodation of cultures. Recognition of diversity. An advanced pluralist democracy. A partnership between citizens and State. A balance that promotes individual freedom and economic prosperity while, at the same time, sharing risks and benefits" (12–13). Diversity has been accepted as a legitimate part of Canadian identity, and pluralism has had significant impact on Canadian law, culture, health care, and social organization.

Multiculturalism has and will continue to affect Canada's health care system, the training and supply of health professionals, and the way that medicine is practised and understood. Some noteworthy examples of this impact include the following: (1) Canada's Indigenous population has a long and distinguished medical tradition that remains viable; (2) immigrant medical practices, such as those associated with Traditional Chinese Medicine or Ayurveda, are offered by a large pool of dedicated practitioners in North America, and all tend to move away from a singular biomedical model of practice (Eisenberg et al., 1993; Frawley, 1990; Williams, 1980); (3) immigration has brought thousands of doctors to our shores, all of whom were trained in environments very different from Canada's, yet many of whom want to practise here and are needed (Hryniuk, 1992); (4) alternative and complementary forms of medicine, often derived from other cultural systems, are increasingly being used by patients to deal with conditions that do not respond well to Western treatments (Burton Goldberg Group, 1995); (5) the biomedical model has now circled the globe, spawning a number of mixed medical traditions (e.g., Cuba), but Canada has not quickly adapted to this hybridity (Alvides, 2000); (6) market demand has brought about a several billion-dollar-a-year industry for over-the-counter therapies and alternate systems of healing (Tisserand, 1987); and (7) there is increasing awareness that culture and ethnicity are critical factors in medical care, such as response to pharmaceutical treatment (Frackiewicz, Sramek, Herrera, Kurtz, & Cutler, 1997). These issues signify that Canadian society, its medical culture, and classical biomedicine are already dealing with cultural issues in very overt and direct ways. This reality has to be engaged and integrated into a larger pattern of Canada's health care understanding.

CULTURE AND ITS CONTEXTS

Every person lives within two contexts—the physical and the social/cultural. Culture was identified as foundational by early anthropologists and was first articulated by E.B. Tylor as "that complex whole which includes knowledge, belief, art, morals, law, custom, and any other capabilities and habits acquired by man as a member of society" (Tylor, 1871, vol. 1, p. 1.). Subsequently, as many as 164 different meanings have been attached to the concept, with the result that identifying the specific context helps determine the meanings assigned (Kroeber & Kluckhohn, 1952). In general, the concept of culture has functioned as a scientific abstraction to identify the basic elements of human life in its social form. Much of social science in the West deals with the analysis of component parts of culture and is itself dependent upon the human ability to assign symbolic meanings to words and speech patterns. In ordinary speech, we assign a bewildering array of activities and meanings to culture, and it is evident that the strength of regional and local expressions militates against associating any universal meaning with the word.

Different cultures use different explanatory models of illness. There are a number of problems with applying the Western medical model in a multicultural setting. Different ethnic groups express illness symptoms in different ways. Western societies have adopted the biomedical basis of disease, which uses an internal locus of control: individuals determine their own fate through actions. In non-Western cultures, health is a constant state of balance between health and illness, even in the absence of symptoms. In this case, the locus of control is external; events are determined by fate. Furthermore, cultural explanations of illness often have implications that are not completely rational or scientific. They may provide explanations that are contrary to what is generally accepted in other cultures or by others in their own culture. Once these views take root in a multicultural society like Canada, they take on a life of their own and become part of the environment within which medicine is practised. Moreover, cultural beliefs determine the perceived importance of symptoms, the subsequent use of resources, and even decisions about how to treat individual patients. Obviously, the study of culture and Western medicine has the potential to generate much controversy.

BIOMEDICAL CULTURE

Let us consider the medical context for the concept of "culture." Traditionally, the most predominant meaning of culture in medicine has dealt with the growth of micro-organisms in a nutrient-rich medium. Such specificity strongly aligns medicine with the science that has dominated the field in the past 100 years. The *biomedical model* of illness has been the basis of modern Western medicine for the past century. Originated by Rudolf Virchow in 1847, the model focuses on physical processes and maintains that all disease stems from cellular abnormalities. The model assumes that illness has a single underlying pathological cause and removal of the pathology will result in a cure (Wade & Halligan, 2004). While the biomedical model has provided a sound framework for understanding and treating disease, and has been the foundation for many advances in medicine during the twentieth century, it is reductionist. It regards the mind and body as being independent, places the locus of responsibility for a person's health on health professionals, and assumes that patient outcomes are determined by access to health professionals and medical care (DeWalt & Pincus, 2003). According to the biomedical model, the patient has limited responsibility for his or her health. This model is rooted in a very simplistic notion of the relation between the mind and body, and does not take into account the influence of psychological or social factors on health. It is generally regarded as not adequate in this day and age for both the scientific tasks and the social responsibilities of medicine. Hence, the World Health Organization definition of health—"health is a state of complete physical, mental, and social well-being and not merely the absence of disease or infirmity" (1946)—extends beyond the physical and biological basis of disease to include the social and psychological determinants of health.

As science evolved from an analytic, reductionistic, and specialized approach to become more contextual and cross-disciplinary, George Engel advanced the *biopsychosocial model* of health and illness (1977). This model recognizes the influence of not only biological, but also psychological (beliefs, relationships, stress) and sociological (social class, poverty, diet, pollution) factors on health. This model shifted the focus from disease to health, and thus medicine has managed to shape itself around some of the abiding themes of the human condition—death, disease, well-being, moral rectitude and ethics, social control, and resource allocation.

More philosophically perhaps, Western biomedicine has come to realize that it, too, is the result of a certain kind of cultural practice—a cultural practice that seems to disregard the very person medicine was developed to assist, as well as quality of life and suffering issues. Indeed, the globalization of medicine has not established health equality nor fostered more uniformity (Farmer, 2000; Edgerton, 1992). What it, in conjunction with economic growth, has in fact done has been to foster diverse cultural developments even in the perception of what medicine should be doing, who should receive it, and who should pay. These discussions are now part of biomedicine's culture.

GLOBALIZATION, CULTURE, AND MEDICINE
Medical practice today operates within a global paradigm, with contributions to its tradition coming from all over the world. Health professionals continue to be trained as if medicine were a Western system without much

conscious attempt to acknowledge that the very designation "Western" arises out of a cultural mindset. Because Europe passed on and developed this distinctive form of medicine, which then became dominant in the world, it is often held that biomedicine is Western. The global success of biomedicine relied in some real sense upon the foundations of colonialism. Indeed, biomedicine has to be one of the most productive systems transferred to other cultures around the globe. Many countries incorporated biomedicine into their societies while retaining some aspects of earlier systems. These are usually designated "folk medicine." The global practice of medicine thus has various kinds of medical traditions interacting with biomedicine. Interestingly, the globalization of biomedicine has not reduced the power of local traditions but has sparked attempts to retain the local and the folk as "more traditional," or even more "human."

The globalization of language has also taken place. The predominance of English in international communications, and certainly in the scientific and medical field, has been growing steadily since World War II. Regardless of the linguistic capabilities of many immigrants to Canada, the health sector is dominated by English outside Quebec; thus immigrants with other language capabilities are often faced with major barriers. Great numbers are unable to function meaningfully in the local English idiom, to say nothing of health literacy demands. While globalization may have broken down national borders, it has not adequately provided the tools for communication on an international scale. An interesting feature of this global language phenomenon is that the more English becomes the *lingua franca* of international business and science, the more it is resisted at the local and traditional level. Local languages deemed to be dying are being resurrected and strengthened (e.g., Welsh and Gaelic). This means that, while the health care professional might be trained in English and might research very well in that language, a considerable part of his or her patient base is not comfortable with that expertise. A crucial challenge for health care in Canada is to deliver services to an increasingly multilingual population whose knowledge of either official language may be only rudimentary.

TOPICS AT THE INTERFACE OF CULTURE AND MEDICINE

The collection of studies in this book reflects many key issues that are at the interface of culture and medicine in Canadian society today. The chapters represent a selected and partial focus on the broad topic of culture and medicine. These were selected on the basis of availability and their alignment to the general topic of culture and medicine. The book is intended to serve as a catalyst for further research and discussion, rather than an exhaustive presentation of related issues.

The book is divided into four discrete parts, each addressing distinctly different types of interfaces between culture and medicine. Part I deals with end-of-life and palliative care. Part II addresses cultural and systemic issues encountered by international medical graduates as they negotiate the nuances of the Canadian educational and health care systems. In part III, the crucial issue of language, communication, and cultural competence is presented. Part IV examines Aboriginal and ethnic traditions related to health and medical care. The topics presented herein will be of interest and relevance to health professionals, medical educators, medical sociologists, anthropologists, geographers, and health policy groups.

In part I, the overriding theme is cultural issues that intersect with medical care at the end of life. Themes of end-of-life and palliative care—who provides it, what configuration it might take, and the role of tradition in defining it—are uppermost. Palliative care is a relatively recent addition to the health care world. Of the many vagaries of human experience, it is the confrontation with the end of life that brings into focus the local and the traditional. The continuities provided by traditional ways bring comfort and stability at the end of life's journey. The three chapters that make up this section highlight the tenacity and significance of the local and "folk" in culture in Alberta, from the continuing influence of traditional religious perceptions among Muslims to the role of traditional culture among Aboriginal peoples.

Immigrants who want to continue their medical careers face significant hurdles in Canada. Part II explores the health care and education system hurdles and cultural assimilation challenges that international medical graduates (IMGs) encounter in integrating into the medical workforce in Canada. The Canadian health care system is another culture for IMGs and they must learn how to negotiate its pitfalls and gain insight into its dynamic in order to succeed. The first and last chapters in this section portray the human face of the journey of IMGs in interacting with and integrating into Canada's health care system. The second chapter describes the procedure of integration within the medical education system. The third chapter delineates the socio-cultural characteristics of those IMGs who were successful in securing a residency position in Alberta.

Part III stresses the cultural nexus of language and cultural competence in medical care. Often in one-on-one encounters between patient and health care provider, communication is the solid ground upon which the patient–provider relationship and treatment decisions are built. Moreover, when caring for diverse patient populations, cultural sensitivity is key to effective communication. What if language is a barrier to accessing health services for patients? What happens if the patient loses the ability to communicate? What if the physician speaks in a language so remote and jargon-laden that only his or her peers understand? What if the physician is not proficient in the language? While English has become the language of science and international medicine, should it be the language of medical service? The first two chapters in this section explore various aspects of communication, and particularly of language. The third chapter examines cultural competence of health professionals in four cultural/ethnic communities in northern Alberta and stresses the need for culturally sensitive training for health professionals.

Part IV presents cultural perspectives on health and health practices in our multicultural society. Canada is now more diverse than at any time in our history. What happens when different cultural traditions interact with Western medicine? How does this affect access to and utilization of health services, the provider–patient relationship, and decisions about treatment and care? How do we deal with this multilingual, multicultural reality? Of the four chapters in this section, two focus on Aboriginal peoples, a group that, as a whole, have not benefitted greatly from Canada's health care system. Indeed, the federal government's own yardstick recognizes how poorly Aboriginal health has responded to it (Health Canada, 2003). If Canada's health system is to be inclusive and universal, it has to find a way to bridge this serious gap. This situation is indicative of a deeper issue. It will not do to regard minority groups as somehow peripheral to the health care system; with the nature of Canada now dramatically multicultural, we no longer have that luxury. These chapters demonstrate how very simple our perceptions of medicine have been to this point in time. As we move forward in health care, we need to develop effective intercultural skills, including an awareness of diverse cultural beliefs and practices, and a respect for differences, tolerance, understanding, and flexibility.

We attempt in this collection to address, through the variety of topics, the interface between culture and medicine, and to probe why this is necessary. No claim to completeness can be made in this discourse. Given the changing situation, it is evident that many such studies should follow in its wake. Obviously Canada cannot be free of the influences of the new globalization that is sweeping so much before it. What is essential is that the gatekeepers of culture and medicine be aware of these movements and position Canadian medicine and culture in such a way that it participates vigorously in shaping the new realities of the twenty-first century.

REFERENCES

Alvides, J.H. (2000). Programa nacional de medicina tradicional y natural. In D. Young (Ed.), *Medicina traditional y natural en Cuba* (pp. 5–40). Edmonton: Centre for the Cross-Cultural Study of Health and Healing, University of Alberta.

Burton Golberg Group. (1993–1995). *Alternative medicine: The definitive guide.* Fife, WA: Future Medicine.

Chrétien, Jean. (1999). Address by Jean Chrétien. *Publius: The Journal of Federalism, 29(4),* 11–14.

DeWalt, D.A., & Pincus, T. (2003). The legacies of Rudolf Virchow: Cellular medicine in the 20th century and social medicine in the 21st century. *Israel Medical Association Journal, 5(6),* 395–97.

Edgerton, R.B. (1992). *Sick societies: Challenging the myth of primitive harmony.* New York: Simon & Schuster.

Eisenberg, D.M., Kessler, R.C., Foster, C., Norlock, F.E., Calkins, D.R., & Delbanco, T.L. (1993). Unconventional medicine in the United States: Prevalence, costs, and patterns of use. *New England Journal of Medicine, 328(4),* 246–52.

Engel, G.L. (1977). The need for a new medical model: A challenge for biomedicine. *Science, 196(4286),* 129–36.

Farmer, P. (2000). *Infections and inequalities: The modern plagues.* Berkeley: University of California Press.

Frackiewicz, E.J., Sramek, J.J., Herrera, J.M., Kurtz, N.M., & Cutler, N.R. (1997). Ethnicity and antipsychotic response. *Annals of Pharmacotherapy, 31(11),* 1360–69.

Frawley, D. (1990). *Ayurvedic healing.* Salt Lake City: Morson.

Health Canada. (2003, March). *A statistical profile on the health of First Nations in Canada.* Ottawa: Health Canada.

Hryniuk, S. (1992). *20 years of multiculturalism.* Winnipeg: St. John's College Press.

Kroeber, A.L., & Kluckhohn, C. (1952). *Culture: A critical review of concepts and definitions.* New York: Random House.

Statistics Canada. (2007a). Immigrant population by place of birth, by province and territory (2006 Census) (Manitoba, Saskatchewan, Alberta, British Columbia). Accessed October 25, 2008, at http://www40.statcan.ca/l01/cst01/demo34c-eng.htm

————. (2007b). Population by mother tongue, by province and territory (2006 Census) (Manitoba, Saskatchewan, Alberta, British Columbia). Accessed October 25, 2008, at http://www40.statcan.ca/l01/cst01/demo11c-eng.htm

Tisserand, R.B. (1987). *The art of aromatherapy*. Rochester, VT: Destiny.

Tylor, Edward B. (1871). *Primitive culture* (7th ed., 2 vols). New York: Brentano's.

Wade, D.T., & Halligan, P.W. (2004). Do biomedical models of illness make for good healthcare systems? *British Medical Journal, 329(7479)*, 1398–1401.

Williams, R. (1980). *Biochemical individuality*. Austin: University of Texas Press.

World Health Organization. Preamble to the Constitution of the World Health Organization as adopted by the International Health Conference, New York, June 19–22, 1946; signed on July 22, 1946 by the representatives of 61 states (Official Records of the World Health Organization, no. 2, p. 100) and entered into force on April 7, 1948. Accessed July 14, 2008, at http://www.who.int/about/definition/en/print.html

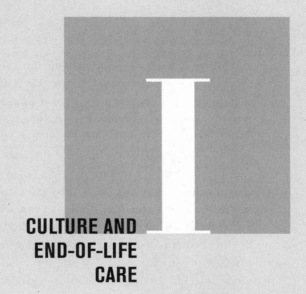

I

**CULTURE AND
END-OF-LIFE
CARE**

OVERVIEW

In Canada, distinct ethnic/cultural views about illness and death coexist in parallel with the Western biomedical culture that is dominant within the health care system. A substantial precentage of Canadians die in hospital; thus end-of-life care has largely moved into the hands of professionals. One would assume, therefore, that the culture established by these institutions would dominate this period of the life cycle at the level of the individual. The studies herein challenge this supposition. There are diverse cultural differences in end-of-life and palliative care, and community views have influenced policy in this area. The studies in this section illustrate that not only do culture and medicine have considerable interaction and inter-connection in northern Alberta, but also cultural difference continues to play an effective role in the provision of care at the end of life.

In the first chapter, "Seeking an Understanding of Aboriginal Culture: A Systematic Review of Aboriginal End-of-Life Care Needs and Preferences," Donna Wilson, Sam Sheps, Roger Thomas, and Margaret Brown summarize how distinctive Aboriginal beliefs and cultural orientations influence attitudes toward death and end-of-life care. Whereas Aboriginals have a preference for the natural and a general acceptance of the situation of impending death, non-Aboriginals tend to fear death. Aboriginals search for meaning as to *why* the disease affects the body rather than *how* the disease affects the body. Aboriginal people tend to avoid decisions about the end of life and prefer care to be delivered in the home community rather than in institutions. These beliefs, perspectives, values, and ethical systems challenge Canadian medical practices in areas of living wills and directives, interventions at the end of life, culturally appropriate communication, and institutional deaths. Issues of communication, differing ideology, and the long-term distrust of mainstream Western culture by Aboriginal groups have contributed to a preference by many Aboriginals to deal with traditional healers instead of Western health professionals. Hence, even where

Western protocols mediate Aboriginal culture, the overall Aboriginal perspective is that Aboriginal culture will maintain the end of life under its own jurisdiction. This underlines the importance of elevating culture as a significant factor in providing end-of-life care and points to greater involvement of culture as a factor in health care policy and the delivery of health services.

The findings of the study on the "Impact of Cultural/Ethnic Perspectives on Dementia and End-of-Life Care in Five Communities in Northern Alberta" present challenges to the biomedical model from varying ethnic and cultural perspectives. Study of the Bigstone Cree in Wabasca, Mandarin- and Cantonese-speaking Chinese in Edmonton, Lebanese Muslims in Lac La Biche, and the francophone community in the Peace Country Health Region indicates that culture plays a role in recognizing, defining, and providing dementia care, and influences end-of-life perception. Cultural values influence the full disclosure of the severity of illness, the use of support services in the community, responsibility and payment for providing care, the decision-making process within the family structure at the end of life, the creation of living wills, appointment of legal guardians, and decisions about resuscitation and life support. Cultural attitudes both shape and frame the role that the health care system plays. The study reveals that variability exists within and between cultural communities on dementia and end-of-life health care issues, and suggests that the evaluation of cultural norms is a pressing issue across Canada in both health service delivery and training of health professionals.

A cultural shift from the traditional biomedical model of providing palliative care services to that of a community-based/community-oriented model is described by Kyle Whitfield and Allison Williams in "Growing Palliative Care: The Story of Alberta." It demonstrates how a culture of community-based care at the level of the population has influenced both policy issues and the delivery of palliative care services in Alberta. In this instance, culture refers to overall societal values and beliefs that are not specific to any one ethnic group. The result has been the integration of home care, long-term care, and community-based services, thus creating some consistency between clinical, cultural, and ethical standards for palliative care services in Alberta.

SEEKING AN
UNDERSTANDING OF
ABORIGINAL CULTURE

A SYSTEMATIC REVIEW OF
ABORIGINAL END-OF-LIFE CARE
NEEDS AND PREFERENCES

Donna M. Wilson RN, PhD

Sam Sheps MD, MSc

Roger Thomas MD, PhD

Margaret Brown MSc

INTRODUCTION

Aboriginal persons have cultural traditions, values, and ethical systems that are distinct from "mainstream" society, with distinctions between and among the many different First Nations groups also to be expected. These extend to conceptions of health and illness generally and thus end-of-life issues specifically. However, Aboriginal groups are often considered homogenous or similar with regard to their needs and interests (Ross, 1992). Aboriginal persons, including North American Indians, Métis, and Inuit, comprise 4.4% of the total population in Canada (Statistics Canada, n.d.). Higher levels of ill health and poverty are among the many problems that show that Aboriginal persons in Canada are disadvantaged relative to the general Canadian population (Royal Commission on Aboriginal Peoples [RCAP], 1996). Reports similarly reveal that this disadvantage exists in countries beyond Canada. Important changes are occurring, however, including growing respect for cultural differences.

Although the number of Aboriginal Canadians living in urban areas now exceeds those residing in rural areas, this rural–urban shift has not translated into higher rates of health and well-being, nor does it appear to have increased access to health care (RCAP, 1996). Cultural and traditional differences, along with socio-economic status and many other factors, are now known to influence hospitalization and other health service utilization rates. Health care diagnoses, treatment decisions, and thus health care treatments also differ as a result of these differences. All accounts consistently reveal that Aboriginal persons die at a younger age than non-Aboriginals. This is one of the few widely known facts about death and dying as it affects Aboriginal persons. Although much attention to the provision of effective and appropriate end-of-life care has been evident since the mid-1970s, when palliative care was first initiated as a distinct and necessary health service, culturally appropriate end-of-life care for Aboriginal persons remains largely unexplored. End-of-life care for Aboriginal persons needs to be based on an understanding and appreciation of distinct Aboriginal perspectives on death and dying. To this end, a literature search was conducted to find relevant original research articles for a systematic review and consolidation of the information they contain; this information was augmented by monographs, policy statements, and other grey literature. The findings of this review offer insight into ways of enhancing the development and provision of Aboriginal end-of-life care. In short, this review sought to identify appropriate end-of-life care for Aboriginal persons.

METHODS

In 2003 and again in 2007, a literature search was performed using nine key library databases: EMBASE, MEDLINE, CINAHL®, Psychinfo, Educational Resources Information Centre (ERICSM), Healthstar, Sociological Abstracts, Cochrane, and AHMED. This search was completed by using the following terms: "hospice," "dying," and "terminal care." These terms were subsequently combined with the following terms: "Aboriginal," "Native," "Indigenous," "First Nation," "Indian," and "research." As the initial 2003 search yielded only two potential English-language research articles for review, the reference lists of these articles were searched for additional research articles. Three more articles that met the inclusion criteria were found. Given the low number of articles and the fact that all were published in peer-reviewed journals, all five were systematically reviewed. A content analysis of the information contained in these articles, undertaken in keeping with standard practices of qualitative data coding and categorization, revealed three themes: (a) substantial differences between Aboriginal persons and mainstream populations need to be recognized, (b) major barriers to communication exist, and (c) a long-standing historical basis for distrust is clearly present and must be accounted for. The 2007 search revealed three additional research articles for review. These articles reinforced and contributed to one or more of the three themes.

Grey literature (i.e., monographs, reviews, policy statements, and non-research articles) on Aboriginal end-of-life care was also sought in 2003 and 2007 to augment the scant amount of research-based information. This search was conducted using the nine aforementioned databases and the First Nations Periodical Index, as well as the World Wide Web. Only a small fraction of the many hits, however, were found to deal specifically with Aboriginal end-of-life care. A limited amount of grey literature (i.e., primarily opinion and experience-oriented articles) was considered informative following a manual analysis of abstracts and full papers. Among these were key documents, such as a book on Aboriginal peoples and their culture by Ross (1992), the report of the Royal Commission on Aboriginal Peoples (1996), a Canadian booklet on end-of-life care that has a chapter on Aboriginal health and end-of-life issues (Fisher, Ross, & MacLean, 2000), two editions of a thanatology book, each having a chapter on early (pre-European and post-European arrival) Canadian deaths and burial customs (Northcott & Wilson, 2001, 2008), and a relatively small number of Canadian or international opinion articles, such as a commentary on end-of-life issues affecting American Indians (Hampton & Castro, 2005).

RESULTS

Substantial Differences Between Aboriginal and Mainstream Populations Need to be Recognized

Differences between Aboriginal and mainstream populations were the focus of six research articles (Campbell, 1989; Hepburn & Reed, 1995; McGrath, 2000, 2007; Willis, 1999; Zebel, 2004). Campbell (1989) explored differences between Aboriginal and mainstream society with respect to their historical and current socio-economic status, approach toward and understanding of health and wellness, and access to health care services. A key finding of this study was that Aboriginal persons tend to search for meaning as to why the disease affects the body, rather than the mechanisms of how the disease affects the body. Campbell indicated that many

Aboriginal persons prefer to deal with traditional healers instead of (or perhaps in conjunction with) modern health care professionals. In addition to the historical and current effects of poverty on health status, Campbell noted that Aboriginal persons' ability to access or develop necessary health services was limited if not hindered by a "myriad of complex rules and governmental regulations" (p. 13). In order to be effective, not only should health services be grounded in Aboriginal culture, but they should also be shaped to fit the needs of differing Aboriginal groups. Campbell indicated that it is imperative to learn and appreciate the·needs of Aboriginal persons with respect to their physical, emotional, and spiritual well-being. In particular, the cultural approaches to and the cultural meanings of grief need to be understood for appropriate care to be extended to the families of terminally ill and dying Aboriginal persons.

Zebek (1994) surveyed family physicians in British Columbia about the use of traditional medicines by their Aboriginal patients, as well as the physician's tolerance of and understanding of these traditional therapies. Zebek found that many physicians had difficulty in being able to determine the health risks and benefits associated with traditional medicines; but physicians were typically accepting of the use of traditional medicines for palliative care purposes. Many physicians, however, were reluctant to develop collaborations with traditional Native healers due to financial, ideological, legal, and philosophical barriers.

After examining the ethical and clinical issues related to end-of-life decision-making affecting elderly Native Americans through a review of literature and interviews of health care providers (i.e., physicians, nurses, social workers, and administrators), Hepburn and Reed (1995) reported that it was essential to understand that significant differences may exist in the way in which Aboriginal groups versus other ethnic and cultural groups approach end-of-life decisions. Furthermore, they noted that there may be major differences across individual Native American groups, and thus a need to assess the cultural and experiential background of each group. The framework of beliefs underlying such decisions may also be significantly different. It also must be recognized that the right of the Aboriginal person to choose for him or herself is strongly and widely held, with the social structures of most Aboriginal groups operating to reinforce and protect this right. Thus, once an individual makes a decision, the family and/or tribal group will typically be supportive of that decision (Hepburn & Reed

1995). In addition, Native American elders, although the most impoverished of all ethnic elderly cohorts, are honoured in Native American groups for having a very strongly held belief in personal autonomy. This respect for personal autonomy is reflected in another key Aboriginal value, "preference for the natural" (p. 105): a preference that means they accept their impending death, as it is "expected and unavoidable. Their decisions, in these circumstances, are in harmony with the larger cycles of life and are taken matter-of-factly and are not seen as great struggles" (p. 105). As elders and their families accept the end of life as unavoidable, they tend to avoid making decisions about end-of-life care, such as those around withholding or withdrawing life-supporting technologies. In the case of patient incompetence, the family gathers, discusses, and accepts the situation of impending death. However, this is often a process that does not fit well with the "urgent" decisions that non-Aboriginal health care professionals feel need to be made. One of the key cultural issues noted in Hepburn and Reed's report (1995) was that the Native American culture is oriented to the present, and that time is perceived as circular rather than as linear—in keeping with their cultural orientation to the "cycles" of life. Consequently, conversations about future-oriented decisions may be outside an Aboriginal person's ordinary paradigm of how one understands and behaves in time. Hepburn and Reed recommended the following guidelines to facilitate more effective communication between health care providers and Aboriginal persons: (i) be clear about the goal of the process; (ii) develop structures that permit unstructured conversation; (iii) assess and be sensitive to the cultural situation of the elder; (iv) be committed to communication; (v) use interpreters when needed; (vi) recognize the elder's family and group; (vii) be prepared to attend to the spiritual and physical well-being of the elder; and (viii) let spokespersons emerge.

Willis's (1999) study of a remote tribe living in central Australia—the Pitjantjatjara Aboriginal people—focused on three areas of interest to the researcher: their preference for dying in their "home" country, their preference for the provision of palliative care through matrilineal kin structures, and the need to overcome difficulties in providing health care in remote areas. Dying was found to be one aspect of living, with dying thus "culturally mediated," as it was an inevitable structural component of life, one clearly that has been lost in Western health care institutions. Willis concluded that simple changes from the way palliative care is normally delivered, since this care was conceived in a different culture, will not automatically make palliative care more appropriate for Aboriginal persons. Instead, care for these persons must be based on their culture, particularly as they have a "culture of dying" (p. 423) that must be understood for appropriate Aboriginal palliative care planning and delivery.

McGrath (2000) also reported on a distinct aspect of Australian Aboriginal culture, as noted among Aboriginal persons living in the Northern Territory of Australia. In the face of disease, these persons search for meaning as to why the disease affects the body, not the mechanisms for how the disease affects the body. Moreover, McGrath found that when health professionals tell the truth about not knowing why the disease affects the body, anger and frustration are experienced among Aboriginal persons. Thus, since these Aboriginal persons may appoint blame when death occurs, Aboriginal health care workers and even family members may be reluctant to become involved near the time of death for fear of being blamed. However, regardless of how or why death occurs, McGrath found that death is considered an everyday part of life, and dying Aboriginal persons typically want to die at home where they feel they belong. Most families also want their family member to die at home, although some families may be reluctant to accept them as they do not have the resources to care for them and do not wish to be held responsible for the death. Families also may not want it to be known that their family structure has broken down through the death of a key family member, such as an elder. In short, McGrath indicates that understanding these and other cultural dynamics is critical for successfully initiating and maintaining palliative care programs for Aboriginal clients.

A more recent Australian study by McGrath (2007) revealed substantial differences between Aboriginal and non-Aboriginal persons with regard to end-of-life care preferences. This qualitative study emphasized the importance for Aboriginals of dying at home as it was conceptualized as their being connected to the land and their family. Dying at home also permitted passing on sacred knowledge to another family member, ensuring that their animal spirit was able to return to the land after their death, and ensuring that the right family member was involved in their care. It was important for them to be in their rightful "death" country. It was also evident that they did not want to die in a large hospital, even if life-saving or effective comfort-oriented treatment could occur there. Non-Aboriginals alternatively were much more accepting of care in hospitals, as this care could potentially achieve a cure and would also provide considerable comfort during a dying process that was often feared.

Major Barriers to Communication Exist

Five of the reviewed articles focused on communication barriers (Hepburn & Reed, 1995; Kaufert, 1999; Kaufert, Putsch, & Lavallee, 1999; Kitz & Berger, 2004; McGrath, 2000). Among these, McGrath (2000) emphasized that poor communication about health and health care leads to dissatisfaction in any society, and good communication leads to better health outcomes. Communication was thus identified as vital in the provision of health care. McGrath found that more than 70% of Aboriginals speak a language other than English at home, while 25% speak little or no English at all; this language barrier can be partially overcome by cross-cultural teamwork and cultural brokerage—a situation when messages, belief systems, and instructions are exchanged between cultural groups. Translators were also identified as essential.

Kaufert et al.'s (1999) Canadian research team similarly found that interpreters facilitated communication, offered cultural mediation, and allowed the mitigation of ethnocentric perspectives. Bicultural health workers were also considered important for educating and informing health care staff about cultural and linguistic differences. As an alternative method of communication, health care providers who were experienced in caring for Aboriginal persons reported that they frequently used indirect communication to engage older patients in discussions about end-of-life decision-making.

A second article by Kaufert (1999) focused on the findings of interviews of Aboriginal patients who were receiving palliative care in urban Canadian hospitals, as well as the findings from interviews of their families, health care providers, and interpreters. Issues around communication and culture were illustrated through case studies involving three patients. Interpreters were identified as critical in the cultural mediation that occurs when discussions need to focus on cancer diagnosis and prognosis, as well as palliative care options. This cultural mediation needed to respect generational differences, as when the Aboriginal person was older, cultural values prohibited direct communication about death and dying. Younger Aboriginal persons were found instead to wish for more direct and open communication about dying and their care options. Interpreters were thus identified as "brokers" in that they mediated in each care situation where the differing viewpoints of involved persons could create a situation of conflicting cultural and ethical values for guiding end-of-life decisions. These conflicting values were particularly emphasized in the ethical areas of truth-telling and autonomy.

Hepburn and Reed's 1995 study of North American elders also revealed a need for interpreters. This study emphasized that interpreters and health care providers need to recognize and accept the elder's family and cultural group as being important with regard to inclusion in discussions about health and health care. A more recent study, one examining end-of-life and palliative care issues at Indian Health Service facilities in the Albuquerque, New Mexico, area, revealed communication barriers as a prime concern with regard to planning and providing end-of-life care services for Aboriginal persons (Kitz & Berger, 2004). This study, involving chart reviews and interviews of health care providers, showed that although there was an open-door policy in existing care facilities on one reserve that allowed traditional medicines and enhanced family visitation, most of the important communications were neither recorded nor facilitated by organizational policies and care standards. As such, end-of-life care was highly individual and thus subject to many difficulties. Communication about important aspects of end-of-life care might not occur or might not be optimal.

A Long-Standing Historical Basis for Distrust is Clearly Present and Must be Accounted For

The historical basis for Aboriginal persons' current distrust of mainstream society and health care was the focus of two research articles (Campbell, 1989; Hepburn & Reed, 1995). Although only two of the research reports emphasized this historic distrust, the report of the Royal Commission on Aboriginal Peoples (1996) indicates that the impact of initial European contact on Native Americans could be characterized as disastrous. Aboriginal people had little or no immunity against the various infectious diseases introduced by the European settlers, such as influenza, tuberculosis, and smallpox. Infectious diseases were responsible for an approximate 80% decline in Aboriginal populations (RCAP, 1996). Not surprisingly, this history continues to be influential in health care relationships.

Given that even more recent relationships have been based on discrimination, colonization, paternalism, and thus ongoing inequality (Campbell 1989; Hepburn & Reed 1995), Native peoples are naturally suspicious and defensive in their interactions with non-Native health care providers. Consequently, relationships need to be restructured on a more equitable basis reflecting a fundamental understanding of distinct Indigenous traditions, values, and ethical systems.

DISCUSSION AND CONCLUSIONS

As indicated previously, few studies pertinent to building an understanding of culturally appropriate Aboriginal end-of-life care have been undertaken. Bonder, Martin, and Miracle (2001) recommend fact-finding about other cultural groups as an important research undertaking, one of two important methods for enhanced cultural competence in a multicultural society.

Despite the obvious dearth of existing research, this review revealed three themes that are relevant to designing and implementing Aboriginal end-of-life care: (a) substantial differences between Aboriginal persons and mainstream populations need to be recognized and then acted upon, (b) major barriers to communication exist, and (c) a long-standing historical basis for distrust is present and must be accounted for. These themes emphasize that although end-of-life care planning and provision is already complex, given the many challenges associated with dying and with grieving, designing end-of-life care for Aboriginal persons is not a matter that can be simply focused on addressing needs arising at or near the end of life. End-of-life care for Aboriginal persons must instead be based upon the importance of dying and death to Aboriginal persons, as this importance extends into all aspects of Aboriginal life. Campbell (1989) concedes that many of the issues revolving around the delivery of health care of Aboriginal persons will not be solved within the boundaries of health care but rather through social means and mechanisms. For instance, as poverty negatively affects health, raising death rates and reducing age at death, poverty among Aboriginals must be addressed to make premature death and dying less common among Aboriginal peoples. Poverty also needs to be addressed as it reduces the ability of family and friends to provide support to dying persons and to each other. Addressing deficits in the living environment of Aboriginal persons is a related issue. Aboriginals may die far from home communities, in cities and city hospitals that are ill equipped to provide distinctively different, culturally appropriate care. In general, this care needs to be less medically driven and more oriented to the social and spiritual needs of Aboriginals. All such considerations should ultimately serve to strengthen the ability of Aboriginal persons to be self-sufficient, to have self-respect, and to see meaning in death as a part of life; as these are important bases to both a good life and a good death.

Obviously, more rigorous research is needed to further assess the differences between Aboriginal and other cultures, and to determine the feasibility of integrating modern Western and traditional Aboriginal health care practices for appropriate end-of-life care (Hampton & Castro, 2005). In addition, care must be taken not to think that knowledge gained through studying one Aboriginal group can be applied to other Aboriginal groups, nor can it be assumed that acculturation to the dominant culture has occurred among younger Aboriginal persons (Hampton & Castro, 2005) or among Aboriginal persons who live in urban areas.

One clear implication, however, from the existing literature would be that end-of-life care for many Aboriginal groups needs to be focused around providing these services in the home community. This change may be difficult for health care providers who are part of a system of health care that is now largely urbanized, medicalized, specialized, and hospitalized. Palliative care in the home and home community would indeed be essential if culturally appropriate care is to be possible. In fact, it follows from the literature that end-of-life care provided in home communities would be essential to the development of trust between Aboriginal patients and their families, and non-Aboriginal health care providers—that is, services must go the patient and family rather than the patient and family going to the services. This shift would also address the need for a deeper understanding of differing conceptions of time, and appropriateness with regard to clinical decision-making and end-of-life care planning. Decisions and decision-making at home or in home communities can be expected to differ from those occurring in mainstream institutions. Thus differences between Aboriginal and non-Aboriginal cultures may be more clearly highlighted with this shift in end-of-life care location—a necessary awakening, and one that may lead to more discussion and more research.

Based on the available research and grey literature, it is also clear that end-of-life care for Aboriginal persons needs to be designed and provided in a manner that underscores the importance of distinct cultural perspectives (Fisher, Ross, & MacLean, 2000; Northcott & Wilson, 2001; Campbell, 1999; Hepburn & Reed, 1995). Ultimately, respect for Aboriginal culture and traditions is essential. According to Bonder et al., in addition to fact-finding, the second way to achieve cultural competence in a multicultural society is by recognizing that it is "impossible to know all there is about every culture" (2001, p. 38). Instead, they argue, an attitude-centred approach is needed, one which emphasizes the importance of valuing other cultures. This approach's advantage, if combined with ethnographical orientations, is that it offers a practical strategy of learning how to ask and of knowing that it is important to ask about others, as opposed to not realizing the importance of asking about what is appropriate and needed for persons who have a different cultural base (Bonder et al., 2001).

Given that only 0.1% of physicians and nurses practising in Canada are Aboriginal (RCAP, 1996), it is non-Native health care professionals who must seek to offer culturally sensitive care. This quest will require them to become aware of subtleties in the conception of health and illness, and communication differences, as well as the need for fostering cultural rituals when providing end-of-life care (Fisher et al., 2000; Roche, 1994; Hepburn & Reed, 1995). Another major need is to increase the number of Aboriginal health care professionals, particularly those who are educated in palliative care and are thus more comfortable in noticing and resolving end-of-life care issues. These persons may also be more adept at addressing the fact that end-of-life care should be constructed so as to address the varying conditions of First Nations persons who could be living in remote, reserve, or non-reserve (urban) places (Campbell, 1989; Fried, 2000; McGrath, 2000). It is also important for all to act upon the recognition that Aboriginal people ultimately want to take over the responsibility for health, healing, and health care decisions in their own communities (RCAP, 1996).

AUTHORS' NOTE

This chapter is based on a report completed for a study "Integrated End-of-life Care: A Health Canada Synthesis Research Project" funded by Health Canada (#6795–15–2002/4780004). The interpretations and conclusions contained herein are those of the researchers and do not necessarily represent the views of the Government of Canada or Health Canada. Neither the Government of Canada nor Health Canada has expressed an opinion in relation to this study.

Additional researchers contributed actively to the research study: Dr. Stephen Birch (McMaster University), Dr. Lise Fillion (Université Laval), Dr. Janice Kinch (University of Calgary), Dr. Tom Noseworthy (University of Calgary), Mr. David Shepherd (County Durham, England), Dr. Corrine Truman (Capital Health, Alberta), Dr. Christopher Justice (McMaster University), Ms. Karen Leibovici (Edmonton city councillor), Dr. Margaret McAdam (Toronto, Ontario), Ms. Pamela Reid (Nova Scotia Community College), and Dr. Karen Olson (University of Alberta).

REFERENCES

Bonder, B., Martin, L., & Miracle, A. (2001). Achieving cultural competence: The challenge for clients and healthcare workers in a multicultural society. *Generations, 25(1)*, 35–43.

Campbell, G.R. (1989). The changing dimension of Native American health: A critical understanding of contemporary Native American health issues. *American Indian Culture and Research Journal, 13(3 & 4)*, 1–20.

Fried, O. (2000). Providing palliative care for Aboriginal patients. *Australian Family Physician, 29(11)*, 1035–38.

Fisher, R., Ross, M.M., & MacLean, M.J. (Eds.). (2000). *A guide to end-of-life care for seniors*. Health Canada: Minister of Supply and Services.

Hampton J.W., & Castro L. (2005). End-of-life issues for American Indians: A commentary. *Journal of Cancer Education, 20 (Suppl. 1)*, 37–40.

Hepburn, K., & Reed, R. (1995). Ethical and clinical issues with Native-American elders: End-of-life decision-making. *Clinics in Geriatric Medicine, 11(1)*, 97–111.

Kaufert, J.M. (1999). Cultural medication in cancer diagnosis and end-of-life decision making: The experience of Aboriginal patients in Canada. *Anthropology and Medicine, 6(3)*, 404–21.

Kaufert, J.M., Putsch, R.W., & Lavallee, M. (1999). End-of-life decision making among Aboriginal Canadians: Interpretation, mediation, and discord in the communication of "bad news." *Journal of Palliative Care, 15(1)*, 31–38.

Kitz, J., & Berger, L. (2004). End-of-life issues for American Indians/Alaska Natives: Insights from one Indian Health Service area. *Journal of Palliative Medicine, 7(6)*, 830–38.

McGrath, C.L. (2000). Issues influencing the provision of palliative care services to remote Aboriginal communities in the Northern Territory. *Australian Journal of Rural Health, 8*, 47–51.

McGrath, P. (2007). "I don't want to be in that big city; this is my country here": Research findings on Aboriginal peoples' preference to die at home. *Australian Journal of Rural Health, 15*, 264–68.

Northcott, H.C., & Wilson, D.M. (2001). *Dying and death in Canada*. Aurora, ON: Garamond.

———. (2008). *Dying and death in Canada* (2nd ed.). Peterborough, ON: Broadview.

Roche, J. (1994). Creative ritual in a hospice. *Health Progress, 75(10)*, 45–47.

Ross, R. (1992). *Dancing with a ghost: Exploring Indian reality*. Markham, ON: Octopus.

Royal Commission on Aboriginal Peoples. (1996). *Report*. 5 vols. Ottawa: RCAP. Available at http://www.ainc-inac.gc.ca/ap/rrc-eng.asp

Statistics Canada. (n.d.). *Aboriginal peoples of Canada (2001 census)*. Available at http://www12.statcan.ca/english/census01/Products/Analytic/companion/abor/canada.cfm

Willis, J. (1999). Dying in country: Implications of culture in the delivery of palliative care in indigenous Australian communities. *Anthropology and Medicine, 6(3)*, 423–35.

Zebek, E.M. (1994). Traditional native healing: Alternative or adjunct to modern medicine? *Canadian Family Physician, 40*, 1923–31.

TWO

IMPACT OF CULTURAL/ ETHNIC PERSPECTIVES ON DEMENTIA AND END-OF-LIFE CARE IN FIVE COMMUNITIES IN NORTHERN ALBERTA

Earle H. Waugh PhD

Olga Szafran MHSA

Jean A.C. Triscott MD, CCFP, FCFP

INTRODUCTION

The diversification of Canada's population by immigration from all over the world and the considerable growth of Canada's seniors population has necessitated that health care professionals become aware of the cultural perspectives that influence how individuals and families from distinct ethnic groups recognize and process dementia and end-of-life situations. Research shows that ethnic factors can indeed influence perceptions of dementia (Morrow-Howell, Chadiha, Proctor, Hourd-Bryand, & Dore, 1996). The cultural perspective is of critical importance in diagnosis because culture plays a role in defining dementia. Major difficulties reside in the assessment tools used for diagnosis (Torti, Gwyther, Reen, Friedman, & Schulman, 2004), as the majority of diagnostic tests are based on cognitive assessments not validated within various cultural contexts (Iliffe & Manthorpe, 2004). Hence, understanding cultural norms, values, beliefs, and frameworks of the disease would greatly benefit health care professionals working with ethnic groups with dementia (Dilworth-Anderson & Gibson, 2002). The guidelines published by the Canadian Consensus Conference on Dementia recognize the influence of culture on dementia (Patterson et al., 1999).

Cultural and environmental factors may play an important role in the prevalence of dementia. South Asian culture has no name for dementia (Iliffe & Manthorpe, 2004) and certain cultural models of expected old-age behaviour may include dementia symptoms as normal aging (Henderson & Henderson, 2002; Teng, 2002). In a study comparing Japanese and Japanese Americans, there was a significantly lower rate of dementia among the Japanese in Japan (Illiffe & Manthrope, 2004). African-Americans in the United States are reported to have the highest rate of dementia of any ethnic group (Cloutterbuck & Mahoney, 2003).

Some ethnic variations in types of dementia have also been noted. The Cree in Manitoba have a higher incidence of vascular dementia and alcohol dementia compared to Alzheimer's. A Canadian study found that, among the Cree, all dementias accounted for 4.2% of cases and Alzheimer's for 0.5% of cases. In comparison, in English-speaking Canadians all dementias accounted for 4.2% of cases and Alzheimer's for 3% of cases (Hall et al., 2000). There has only been limited research on the mental health of ethnic minority elders (Iliffe & Manthorpe, 2004) and very little research on dementia or dementia caregivers among the Indigenous population of northern America (Henderson & Henderson, 2002; Jervis & Manson, 2002).

Family involvement and responsibilities translate into different perceptions of need for services for families of dementia patients. Family beliefs also influence and impact the use of a supportive service by caregivers of dementia patients (Neufeld, Harrison, Stewart, Hughes, & Spitzer, 2002). Family members, friends, and other informal supports, with or without supplementary assistance from formal services (e.g., home health), provide approximately 70–80% of the care of non-institutionalized frail older persons (Cagney & Agree, 1999).

Language often is a barrier to caregiving. Dementia patients who lose the ability to communicate in their acquired language may find communication with their caregivers difficult (Iliffe & Manthorpe, 2004); caregivers may be unable to accurately communicate informed consent (Kaufert, 1999) due to language difficulties. Family translators may choose not to disclose the extent of the diagnosis to the patient, as cultural values may discourage full disclosure of the severity of the disease (Rosenberg, Leanza, & Seller, 2007).

There is an unprecedented need for Canadian health care providers to respond to an increasing population of dementia sufferers, families, and caregivers in a culturally competent way—considering both the disease and contextual cultural factors. In order to gain a better understanding of the influence of culture on dementia and end-of-life care, we conducted a study to examine how dementia and end-of-life issues are recognized and cared for in five different cultural communities in northern Alberta (Cree, francophone, Mandarin-speaking Chinese, Cantonese-speaking Chinese, and Muslim).

METHODS
Study Design
This study employed elements of participatory research and a modified consensus group process to examine how dementia and end-of-life issues are recognized and cared for in five cultural/ethnic communities in northern Alberta. Consensus groups were used to obtain agreement within each cultural/ethnic community on the group's attitudes and opinions toward issues related to dementia and end-of-life care. Elements of the participatory research process were used to engage each community in the overall development and implementation of the project, the development of culturally specific questionnaires, identification of community members for consensus groups, and the synthesis and interpretation of the study findings.

The study participants included community members 55 years of age or older, belonging to each of five communities in northern Alberta: (1) Bigstone Cree in Wabasca; (2) francophones in the Peace Country Health Region; (3) Cantonese-speaking Chinese in Edmonton; (4) Mandarin-speaking Chinese in Edmonton; and (5) the Lebanese Muslim community in Lac La Biche. All consensus group members were either recent or past immigrants to Canada and were familiar with the cultural values, traditions, and actions of their group.

Participating Communities
Bigstone Cree in Wabasca: The Cree people are perhaps the most widespread of all cultural/language groups of Indigenous peoples in Canada. Depending upon the reading of the historical sources, the Cree migrated

from the east in various waves and were the first Aboriginal group encountered in Hudson Bay in 1682 (Hlady, 1960). There is some evidence that the Cree had come long before the impulses from the fur trade (Russell, 1991). Wabasca, some 123 kilometres north of Edmonton, was an old landing for the missionaries and fur hunters in the early days of western exploration and was a focal point for interaction between the Cree and Europeans (Vandersteene, 1960). Always small in numbers, the small bands and groups of families settled in areas amenable to hunting and fishing around the Wabasca landing. Eventually, the Cree in the region amalgamated into the Bigstone Band and signed Treaty 8 (1899) deeding land to the government in exchange for education and health services (Waugh, 1996). The Bigstone Band is located 300 kilometres north of Edmonton and has a population of approximately 2,300 (Indian and Northern Affairs Canada, 2007). There is widespread resistance among these peoples (and other Aboriginal groups in Canada) to being referred to as an "ethnic group," and we shall honour this perception in this chapter.

Francophones in Peace Country Health Region: The francophone community in the Peace Country Health Region of northwestern Alberta participated in this study. Francophone members from the towns of St. Isadore, Guy, Falher, and MacLennan took part in the consensus group process. French communities have been the bedrock of European immigration to northern Alberta, with several family clusters dating back to the fur-trade period. Although the pressure to assimilate has been great, especially in the early days of English administration, these communities have retained their French character and culture. We worked with the co-ordinator for health services in French in the region to identify francophone individuals to participate in the consensus group process.

Chinese in Edmonton: Edmonton is a metropolitan city with a total population of 927,020 people and a Chinese population of 44,445 (4%) according to the 2001 census (Statistics Canada, 2001). There are two parallel Chinese immigrant communities in Edmonton, one speaking Mandarin, the other Cantonese. We were advised by each of the communities to consider them two distinct communities. While the two groups are not mutually exclusive, there were sufficient differences in migration and type of community to consider them separate groups for the purposes of this study. Chinese immigrants have been present throughout the northern part of the province beginning in the twentieth century; however, since the 1980s, the Chinese population has boomed. Many elderly have come as part of this increasing immigration, often as retired relatives of migrating children. Some of these people understand very little English and rely upon their close relatives for information and translation. We worked with the Edmonton Chinese Lions Club to identify the members for the Cantonese-speaking and Mandarin-speaking Chinese consensus groups.

Lebanese Muslims in Lac La Biche: Muslim immigrants have been part of the complexity of the north from early times, with a Lebanese Muslim presence dating back to the fur trade in northern Alberta. Significant numbers came after the end of the World War II, and many of them settled in Lac La Biche, located 220 kilometres northeast of Edmonton. Muslims in Lac La Biche comprise 6.7% (180 out of 2,670) of the town's total population (Statistics Canada 2006 Census). By comparison, Muslims comprise 2.15% of the population in North America. The Arabic-speaking, Lebanese Muslim community in Lac La Biche is well-organized, with a mosque and cultural components firmly in place. We worked with the Council of the Alkareem Mosque—Lac La Biche Muslim Association to recruit community members for the consensus group. The group insisted that the elderly males of their society reflected the views of both males and females within the community, this being their traditional religious/cultural role. As such, the Muslim consensus group consisted of only male members of the community.

Consensus Group Process

The consensus group process was used to obtain each respective community's consensus response to items on a questionnaire. The process involved a group discussion of 10–20 community members about issues related to dementia and the end of life. It is a participative technique for determining group attitudes and opinions, partway between a focus group and a public meeting, where the participants themselves negotiate the findings (List, 2001). The main difference between consensus groups and focus groups is who decides on the group outcomes. Whereas a consensus group should reach agreement and participants themselves decide on the group outcomes, a focus group is not required to reach a consensus and the facilitator/data analyst decides on the group outcomes through an analytic approach. Our rationale for using the consensus group technique was that group agreement on various issues was desirable in order to determine distinctive differences between cultural groups. As such, a synthetic (rather than analytic) approach was selected.

Each consensus group meeting was led by a community-chosen, bilingual facilitator who was also a member of the respective cultural group. The task of the facilitator was to obtain agreement within the group about the most culturally appropriate response to each question and to record the group response. The consensus group discussion was held in each of the respective communities. The facilitator was also involved in identifying community members who were willing to take part in the consensus group, and later assisted the study team in clarifying any outstanding issues. Consensus groups met one to two times to reach consensus and complete the questionnaire, and each meeting lasted approximately three hours. A total of 65 community members participated in the five consensus groups.

Questionnaires

The study questionnaire addressed specific "dementia-type" and end-of-life cultural issues, such as (1) the meaning of the illness (age vs. disease); (2) family/community values and roles in caregiving; (3) expectation and utilization of health services; (4) end-of-life emphases and expectations; and (5) an invitation to identify lacunae. The questionnaire was individually adapted to be sensitive to each ethno-cultural group. The consensus groups then provided the response that represented their perception of community's view on the issue. Given the area of study, a questionnaire survey of all community members was considered inappropriate, as cultural issues tend to be biased by how (wording and language) the question is asked, and cultural nuances are better addressed in a discussion environment.

After all consensus group processes were completed, the research team met with each facilitator and two community-chosen members to review the consensus responses and confirm their understanding of the community's responses. A number of the questions were similar for all the groups, which enabled comparison between groups. At the request of the francophone community, their questionnaire was translated into French. For the other groups, the questions were translated verbally by the facilitator during the consensus group meeting, if necessary.

RESULTS AND DISCUSSION

Given the topic of this study and the data analysis approach, the challenge of separating findings and discussion became obvious early on. As such, it was deemed that reporting the study findings and concurrently providing a context and/or interpretation for the findings would be the most effective approach to understanding the study results. As such, the results and discussion are presented here in tandem.

Consensus group findings are presented according to the following main themes arising from the data: (1) dementia recognition markers; (2) cultural/religious principles and values and physician consultation; (3) health care responsibility for dementia; (4) caregiving; (5) living wills/legal guardians; (6) resuscitation and end-of-life care; and (7) language. Although there were some variations in responses between groups, with some groups emphasizing issues for their own reasons, there were important uniformities across the groups.

Dementia Recognition

All cultural groups regarded forgetfulness and losing one's way in the elderly as a problem that required critical care immediately. This did not mean that all cultures accepted the medical definition of dementia, as the Bigstone Cree in Wabasca have no word in their vocabulary that corresponds to the medical concept of dementia, and it is not an illness recognized traditionally. The Cantonese-speaking Chinese were reluctant to accept that the illness could be "mental." This is based upon an aversion to accepting "mental illness" in the family line, for social and political reasons.

All cultural groups felt that special treatment is required when the elderly are lethargic or confused, and have problems with medication. When behaviour is marked by lethargy or confusion in areas not noted at an earlier period of the person's life (i.e., unable to find the way home), then all groups accepted that this was a condition that had to be treated. The Bigstone Cree and Chinese groups did not accept that the patient needed to be treated for an "illness," however. Negative incidents of a cognitive nature were generally assigned to the aged; hence, linking cognitive decline to the aging process was accepted by all cultural groups in our study.

Cultural/Religious Principles and Values

Health care professionals sometimes are faced with asking a patient's relatives for assistance when dealing with a case of dementia or when hospital translators are not available. Who has the authority to make decisions in a family structure may not be directly evident even when attempts are made to determine this from those attending the patient. When asked who the health care professional should look to when seeking this authorization, the responses differed between groups. Within the Lebanese Muslim community in Lac La Biche, normally the oldest and closest male blood relative speaks for the incapacitated elderly person, even if a female relative might be emotionally closer to the patient. Among the Cantonese-speaking Chinese group, the oldest son takes on the responsibility for all major health decisions; community members indicated that a strong hierarchical family system persists in Canada, with the emphasis arising out of Confucian values that are the legacy of pre-Communist China. Unlike the Cantonese-speaking Chinese, who were more traditional in their hierarchical perceptions, the Mandarin-speaking Chinese community indicated that consultation was required with all family members, depending on education and economic status. The Mandarin-speaking Chinese also stressed the value of the person as an individual, much the same as Western culture has emphasized. There was reluctance among the Mandarin-speaking Chinese to regard a person as an end-of-life "case," and the community called for more compassion and respect for the elders as a group.

Among the Bigstone Cree in Wabasca, there was continuing belief that the end of life is an engagement with the spirit world, and only ceremonialists or holy people who have access to that world will have insight into the time of death (i.e., not the physician, who has no experience of the spirit world). The health care consequence of this view is that the doctor should not speak about probabilities of death, and health personnel generally should neither discuss life's cessation nor allude to it in attitude, unless the issue is deliberately raised by a close family member. Different strategies may provide another way to deal with a potential death, such as a storytelling circle, where stories addressing death will convey the viewpoint.

Within the francophone community in the Peace Country Health Region, the elderly have strong religious values and beliefs that mediate end-of-life issues. There are obvious differences between the most elderly and their adult children on resuscitation protocols, with middle-aged children of elders stressing the need for the protocols, while the elderly reject them.

Health Care Responsibility

One of the sharpest points of diversion of opinion surfaced around the issue of health care responsibility. There were two areas of keen difference. Among the Muslim and francophone groups, both with strong extended-family orientation, the focus for all aspects of care was the larger "family." This was taken to mean all those who had either a close blood relationship or familial ties. In some sense, the "community" had to be linked to this family network. All aspects of serious care required someone to canvass this larger group on key issues. In the Muslim community of Lac La Biche, generally it was the responsibility of the closest male member to inform and consult with as wide a family circle as possible. For the Cree in Wabasca and for both Chinese groups, the nuclear family made up the first line of responsibility. For the Cree, the nuclear family, understood as the closest relations to the patient, was believed to be initially responsible for these decisions. Once it became clear that the end of life was near, the nuclear family then engaged the community in the rituals and protocols of celebrating the person's life. While the term "nuclear family" may have quite different meanings among the Chinese, all aspects of remembering one's life were a nuclear family responsibility. The family would then engage the community to whom the person was known.

Distinctions were noted regarding who should pay for treatment outside the community. Among Muslims, there was no doubt that the Qur'an had made each family responsible for caring for its elderly. This was so even though the Canadian system provided publicly funded options. In contrast, the francophones in the Peace Country Health Region stressed Canada's universal health care system as the primary institution responsible for providing health services. The Cree in Wabasca insisted that the federal government was responsible, arising out of First Nations' treaties with the Crown.

While the Lebanese Muslim community in Lac La Biche felt that care should be provided in the home, all of the other cultural groups felt that elderly who are at serious risk to themselves or others should be institutionalized. All groups felt it was very unacceptable to move the aged to a home outside the community, except for the Cantonese-speaking Chinese, who indicated that it was somewhat acceptable, depending upon the circumstances.

Caregiving

Consistently, consensus groups indicated that the nuclear family would decide who would care for someone requiring supervision. The groups differed in terms of who would take responsibility for caring for the ill elderly in the home. Both the Lebanese Muslim and Cantonese-speaking Chinese groups believed that the primary responsibility for providing care in the home rested with one individual. Among the Lebanese Muslim group, caring for the ill at home was deemed a religious requirement, and the unmarried daughter accepted this duty as God's will. The Cantonese-speaking Chinese group had strong commitments to ancestral ties, which connected them to a lineage within the spiritual realm, and it was the responsibility of the wife of the eldest son to provide care to ill family members in the home. This was a cultural norm that had long remained standard in the family tradition. Among Mandarin-speaking Chinese, caregiving was much less structured and responsibility for caregiving was determined by a family decision. Who ultimately would provide care might arise out of a family meeting, at which point the decision would be made about caregiving. The Bigstone Cree community insisted that caregiving is an immediate family matter. Who was responsible likely arose from whoever could be freed from his or her work. It was possible that a grandparent might agree to care for someone younger. Among the francophones in the Peace Country Health Region, it was the norm that the closest family member would be responsible, although he or she might arrange with another relative to assist. All groups wanted more support for care in the home because they felt a loyalty and commitment to the aged, who in many cases had expended a great deal of effort on their behalf at some point in their lives. If it were evident that the patient was too advanced for home care, then decisions about institutionalizing the patient would be made.

Notable differences appeared among the groups on the issue of payment for caregiving. The Bigstone Cree Nation community felt strongly that, if a family member took up the caregiving role, that member should be funded by the government as part of its treaty obligations. The Lebanese Muslim group considered that it was a specific family obligation to be paid by the family involved; the Chinese community felt that the health care system should pay. Both Chinese groups felt that the family had the responsibility to ensure that their elders had the very best care, with the Cantonese-speaking Chinese affirming that the eldest son ultimately had to make any final decision on family expenditures for elder well-being and treatment. Mandarin speakers, with less extended family in Canada to support them, left decision-making to the nearest next-of-kin. Both groups held that the financial responsibility for elder care rested with the government. Some felt that the family could ultimately be responsible for payment, but that public resources should be utilized to assist them; others held that it would have to be the responsibility of the government to provide a health care worker to care for the aged, if necessary. The francophone group generally held to the accepted practice that held the nuclear family financially responsible, with government only being involved if the family could not manage financially.

Living Wills and Legal Guardians

The responses to the question about whether members of the group made living wills or personal directives appeared to be influenced by cultural identity. Members of the Bigstone Cree community indicated that no forward planning of living wills or personal directives had ever been part of their tradition. The Mandarin-speaking Chinese and Lebanese Muslim communities indicated that they rarely did this, usually for personal reasons. However, the Cantonese-speaking community sometimes signed personal directive cards, indicating that the concept, at the very least, had some impact within their group. The francophone group was far more likely to have signed such as a directive, with the consensus group indicating that they "often" did so.

There were also important differences between the groups regarding the issue of legal guardians. In terms of how often members appoint legal guardians, both Mandarin-speaking Chinese and Bigstone Cree communities indicated that their members never signed such a document, while the Cantonese-speaking Chinese and Lebanese Muslim community members did so rarely. In terms of personal directives, the francophone group indicated that members often signed such legal documents.

Resuscitation and End-of-Life Care

When questioned on the amounts and types of intervention at the end of life, the Lebanese Muslim community stressed that as much technology as possible should be used to keep a person alive on life support, but that caution should be used with extraordinary means for resuscitation. The Cantonese- and Mandarin-speaking Chinese communities strongly approved of active medical intervention in end-of-life care, since this was an expression of the family's dedication to their presence. Bigstone Cree community members appeared to somewhat approve of medical intervention depending on the individual and amount of suffering involved, but felt that the closest family member could best help the medical team, since that person would know the community values.

All groups felt that an elderly person would want resuscitation if heart or breathing stopped, except for the Bigstone Cree, who would rarely want such resuscitation. The members of the francophone group felt that there should be minimal intervention at the end of life. It was clear that older francophone people felt quite comfortable in their life coming to its normal end, while the younger generation wanted to retain the presence of the older members because of their commitment to French culture and language, cultural strengths that the younger generation felt rather inadequate to sustain.

Language

While the questionnaire did not specifically address the issue of language, all groups indicated that language was of major concern. As noted earlier, the Bigstone Cree have no word for dementia, so conveying information to unilingual Cree speakers that the health care professionals regarded them as having a significant illness would be difficult. Moreover, the Bigstone Cree community felt that it was not the prerogative of health care professionals to diagnose elders with something that was not even part of their conceptual system. Language appeared to be a significant barrier for both Chinese groups in terms of accessing health care and relating to health care workers. The Lebanese Muslim community noted the serious problem they had with the elderly in comprehending English, especially when permission was being sought for medical intervention. The francophone community, in contrast, had been part of Anglo culture for so long that they did not have a problem; most members were thoroughly bilingual. All groups noted that there were circumstances when language was a definite barrier to good health care. Further information on this aspect is found in Jean Triscott's article, entitled "Reflections on Language in the Management of Dementia" (see chapter 9 of this volume).

STUDY LIMITATIONS

The study involved only one specific geographic community within each cultural group; therefore, how representative and generalizable the study findings are is unknown. The assumption was made that the consensus responses from each cultural group reflect the wider community position on each issue, obviously a limitation since communities can harbour diverse opinions on matters of health. Furthermore, while the Lebanese Muslim community stressed that the elderly males reflected the views of both males and females within the community, we consider the lack of female representation in the Muslim consensus group to be a limitation of the study. The francophone people represented in this study were actually spread throughout several communities in the Peace Country Health Region; therefore, the meaning of "community" is flexible in this case.

CONCLUDING SUMMARY

The five Alberta communities revealed a range of cultural/ethnic perspectives on dementia and end-of-life care. While cognitive problems were regarded as an illness of the elderly, not all cultures accepted the medical concept of dementia. The Bigstone Cree did not recognize dementia as an illness, and Cantonese-speaking Chinese were reluctant to accept that dementia can be "mental." Moreover, there were cultural/ethnic differences in terms of whom health care professionals should look to when seeking authority to make decisions in an end-of-life situation. While for Lebanese Muslims, religious beliefs dictated who takes responsibility for providing care in the home of the elderly ill, for Cantonese-speaking Chinese, this responsibility was based on a cultural norm that is rooted in family tradition. For other groups, responsibility for caregiving was based on a family decision. In terms of responsibility for payment for caregiving in the home, Lebanese Muslims considered this to be a family obligation while the Bigstone Cree felt that the government should fund caregiving in the home as part of its treaty obligation. All groups wanted more support for care in the home.

There were significant differences among the groups with respect to making living wills and appointing legal guardians. In contrast to the francophone group, who quite often made willing wills and personal directives, the Bigstone Cree had not made advance preparation in this regard, as this has not been part of their tradition. The francophones reported that they often signed documents appointing legal guardians, whereas the Mandarin-speaking Chinese and Bigstone Cree never did so. Most groups approved of active medical intervention to keep a person alive; however, the Lebanese Muslim group advised caution with extraordinary means of resuscitation and the Bigstone Cree stipulated that this should be done in consultation with the closest family member. All cultural/ethnic groups studied indicated that there were circumstances when language was a barrier to obtaining good quality care for the elderly. An understanding of how various cultural/ethnic groups view end-of-life care and the influence it has on family caregivers and the community will aid in the development of culturally appropriate community services.

AUTHORS' NOTE

This study was funded by the Pallium Project (Phase II under the aegis of the Primary Health Care Transition Fund, Health Canada). The views expressed herein do not necessarily represent the official policies of Health Canada as a major funding provider or the Alberta Cancer Board as administrative hosting authority for the Pallium Project. No competing industry funding was utilized. A special thanks to all the group facilitators and consensus group participants, without whom this study would not be possible. We are grateful to Bunny Bourgeois for administrative assistance on this project.

REFERENCES

Cagney, K.A., & Agree, E.M. (1999). Racial differences in skilled nursing care and home health use: The mediating effects of family structure and social class. *Journal of Gerontology: Social Sciences, 54B(4)*, S223-S236.

Cloutterbuck, J., & Mahoney, D.F. (2003). African American dementia caregivers. *Dementia, 2(2)*, 221–43.

Dilworth-Anderson, P., & Gibson, B.E. (2002). The cultural influence of values, norms, meaning, and perceptions in understanding dementia in ethnic minorities. *Alzheimer Disease and Associated Disorders, 16(2)*, S56–S63.

Hall, K.S., Gao, S., Emsley, C.L., Ogunniyi, A.O., Morgan, O., & Hendrie, H.C. (2000). Community screening interview for dementia (CSI 'D'); Performance in five disparate study sites. *International Journal of Geriatric Psychiatry, 15(6)*, 521–31.

Henderson, J.M., & Henderson, L.C. (2002). Cultural construction of disease: A "supernormal" construct of dementia in an American Indian tribe. *Journal of Cross-Cultural Gerontology, 17(3)*, 197–212.

Hlady, W.M. (1960–61). Indian migrations in Manitoba and the West. *Transactions of the Manitoba Historical Society, ser. 3, 17*, 24–53.

Iliffe, S., & Manthorpe, J. (2004). The debate on ethnicity and dementia: From category fallacy to person-centered care. *Aging & Mental Health, 8(4)*, 283–92.

Indian and Northern Affairs Canada. (2007). Backgrounder—Bigstone Cree Nation and communities of Calling Lake, Chipewyan Lake, Peerless Lake and Trout Lake Agreement-in-Principle. Accessed June 3, 2010, at http://www.ainc-inac.gc.ca/ai/mr/nr/s-d2007/2-2945-bk-eng.asp

Jervis, L.L., & Manson, S.M. (2002). American Indians/Alaska natives and dementia. *Alzheimer Disease & Associated Disorders, 16(2)*, S89–S95.

Kaufert, J.M. (1999). End-of-life decision making among Aboriginal Canadians: Interpretation, mediation, and discord in the communication of "bad news." *Journal of Palliative Care, 15(1)*, 31–38.

List, D. (2001). The consensus group technique in social research. *Field Methods, 13(3)*, 277–90.

Morrow-Howell, N., Chadiha, L.A., Proctor, E.K., Hourd-Bryant, M., & Dore, P. (1996). Racial differences in discharge planning. *Health and Social Work, 21(2)*, 131–39.

Neufeld, A., Harrison, M.J., Stewart, M.J, Hughes, K.D., & Spitzer, D. (2002). Immigrant women: Making connections to community resources for support in family care giving. *Qualitative Health Research, 12(6)*, 751–68.

Patterson, C.J.S., Gauthier, S., Bergman, H., Cohen, C., Freightner, J., Feldman, H., & Hogan, D.B. (1999). The recognition, assessment and management of dementing disorders: Conclusions from the Canadian Consensus Conference on Dementia. *Canadian Medical Association Journal, 160(12 suppl.)*, S1–S15.

Rosenberg, E., Leanza, Y., & Seller, R. (2007, October). *Communication behaviors in physician–interpreter–patient encounters.* Paper presented at North American Primary Care Research Group (NAPCRG) Annual Meeting, Vancouver, BC.

Russell, D.R. (1991). *Eighteenth-century western Cree and their neighbours.* Hull: Canadian Museum of Civilization.

Statistics Canada. (2001). Population by selected ethnic origins, by census metropolitan areas (2001 Census) (Edmonton). Accessed November 28, 2007, at http://www40.statcan.ca/l01/cst01/demo27w.htm?sdi=Edmonton

Statistics Canada. (2006). Community profile for Lac La Biche, Alberta (2006 Census). Accessed November 28, 2007, at: http://www12.statcan.gc.ca/census-recensement/2006/dp-pd/prof/92-591/details/page.cfm?Lang=E&Geo1=CSD&Code1=4812035&Geo2=PR&Code2=48&Data=Count&SearchText=Lac%201a%20Biche&SearchType=Begins&SearchPR=01&B1=All&Custom=

Teng, E.L. (2002). Cultural and educational factors in the diagnosis of dementia. *Alzheimer Disease & Associated Disorders, 16(2)*, S77–S79.

Torti, F.M., Gwyther, L.P., Reed, S.D., Friedman, J.Y., & Schulman, K.A. (2004). A multi-national review of recent trends and reports in dementia caregiver burden. *Alzheimer Disease & Associated Disorders, 18(2)*, 99–109.

Uhlman, R.F, & Larson, E.B. (1991). Effect of education on the Mini-Mental State Examination as a screening test for dementia. *Journal of the American Geriatric Society, 39(9)*, 876–80.

Vandersteene, Roger. (1960). *Wabasca: Dix ans de vie Indienne.* Gemmenich, Belgium: Editions OMI.

Waugh, Earle. (1996). *Dissonant worlds: Roger Vandersteene among the Cree.* Waterloo: Wilfrid Laurier University Press.

THREE

GROWING
PALLIATIVE CARE

THE STORY OF ALBERTA

Kyle Y.T. Whitfield PhD

Allison Williams PhD

INTRODUCTION

Approaches to providing palliative and end-of-life care services in Alberta are changing. A shift is occurring away from a culture that has been led by a traditional biomedical model in the provision of health services and toward a culture that is more community-based and community-oriented. This chapter describes the story of how this cultural shift has influenced policy-related events that have, historically as well as currently, impacted the design and delivery of palliative and end-of-life care services in Alberta. To understand changes in policy processes, a six-stage policy analysis process (Springate-Baginski & Soussan, 2001) is used. The policy and program picture described in each of these six stages is used to broaden the story of the development of palliative and end-of-life care services through time. Policy analysis works as the thread linking each of the six stages outlined.

BACKGROUND: HOW A CULTURE OF COMMUNITY-BASED CARE INFLUENCES PALLIATIVE CARE POLICY PROCESSES IN ALBERTA

A culture of community-based care is influencing palliative care policy processes in Alberta due to substantial directions occurring in the primary care sector, and in palliative and end-of-life care services in particular. Principles of accessible health care (via service integration), community participation, and sustainable collaborative partnerships (Wedel, Grant-Kalischuk, & Patterson, 2007) are playing a strong role in moving this community-based culture forward. Focus is shifting away from hospitals and medical treatment, and toward prevention and health improvement within the community (Romanow, 2002). For example, Pallium, a community-based initiative in Alberta (and Saskatchewan, Manitoba, and the Northwest Territories), has contributed to the creation of a community-focused culture that is improving access to system-linked education and professional development in palliative and end-of-life care for health care professionals and citizen-consumers (Wilson Associates, 2002). At its core is community capacity building.

A culture where community capacity building is a priority is characterized by concepts of empowerment, where enabling processes are used to allow individuals and communities to have more control in their lives and in their environment, according to Julian Rappaport (cited in Minkler, 2005, p. 26). As well, a community capacity-building culture believes that the community itself, rather than outside agencies, is most cognizant of its most important issues and, Marie Nyswander argued, best knows the processes that "start where the people are at" (cited in Minkler, 2005, p. 27), rather than having processes imposed from outside. A culture that focuses on community building is one where processes are used that assist community-based groups to identify common problems or goals, mobilize relevant resources, and develop and implement strategies to reach their collective goals (Minkler & Wallerstein, 2005). A culture where community building is occurring is one where "people who identify themselves as members of a shared community, and their allies in larger systems, engage together in the process of community change" (p. 26). In contrast, a service culture based on a biomedical model assumes that individuals and communities only have deficiency and problems; individuals are seen as service recipients only (McKnight & Kretzmann, 2005; Minkler, 2005, p. 158); health is defined as the absence of disease; and the health system is dominated by doctors (Sprenger, 2005).

Although a culture of community continues to evolve and grow in the realm of palliative and end-of-life care services in Alberta, a broad systematic approach still does not exist (Canadian Institute for Health Information [CIHI], 2007). Alberta is, however, creating and building a culture where there is integration between home, long-term care, and community-based services (CIHI, 2007), where a "good death" culture is fostered (Northcott & Wilson, 2001), and where there is consistency between clinical, cultural, and ethical standards (Field & Cassel, 1997).

METHODOLOGY

To investigate palliative and end-of-life care development in Alberta, two major sources of data were accessed and analyzed: 1) government documents, documents published by community organizations and individuals, and statistical reports; and 2) key informant narratives. The informants are cited in this chapter according to codes (e.g., AB01, AB02, etc.) to protect confidentiality.

A content analysis and a constant-comparison methodology were used to produce a synthesis of the trends, events, and policy developments in palliative and end-of-life care in Alberta, over time. The policy map or timeline (table 1) illustrates our interpretations of the historical progression of policy development and events; upon their completion, we compared our documentation accounts to those of our key informants.

Individual, semi-structured key informant interviews took place with seven informants (N = 7). Six of the seven interviews were conducted over the telephone while the other took place face-to-face. The average length of time of the interviews ranged from 1 to 1.5 hours. Interviewees represented three main constituent groups: clinical (medical sector); government; and health consulting. Thematic analysis of interview transcripts is therefore limited to those perspectives only. The interviews with these key informants allowed us to verify and/or modify the authenticity of the policy map or timeline. Springate-Baginski and Soussan's (2001, p. 11) six-stage "policy process analysis matrix" was used to guide us through the analysis and to comprehend the policy trends and developments over time in Alberta.

When contacting key informants, a systematic process was used. From a list of potential respondents identified as experts in palliative and end-of-life care in Alberta, initial contact was made via email inviting the individual to participate in the study. If the person replied (via email) stating that he or she was interested in participating in the study, a date and time for a telephone interview was agreed upon. If potential respondents did not respond (via email) after a one-to-two-week period, a second email was sent further requesting their participation. If there still was no response, we followed up with a telephone call approximately one week later. If potential respondents did not respond by that stage, no further contact was made. The snowball technique was also used to further identify potential key informants with similar expertise, that is, at the end of an interview, the key informant was asked to recommend another potential key informant that may consider participating in our study.

Approximately one week prior to the interview, key informants received interview questions (appendix A) and our policy map or timeline of the policy-related events impacting the design and delivery of palliative care services in Alberta. As well, they received a consent form to gain their written consent to participate in the study (to fulfill research ethics approval).

Using this overall process of analysis helped to reveal 1) possible points of complexity in the policy development process; 2) ways in which the policy can, and/or has, affected the lives of the people for whom it is intended; and 3) the "messy business" of policy development, affected by more than the decision-makers. Springate-Baginski and Soussan's strategy (2001) is grounded in reality. It captures innovation and downturns in the policy development process, and targets the links between policy development and the impacts the process has on those whom it is intended to affect. We chose to begin our analysis in the 1970s to coincide with several inaugural developments in palliative and end-of-life care in Canada.

The trajectory of policy and related events impacting design and delivery of palliative and end-of-life care services in Alberta (table 1) is mainly grounded in the documentary analysis and is enhanced by information generated from the key informants. The overall story of palliative and end-of-life care in Alberta, therefore, is generated from the integration and synthesis of the key informant interviews, and from the documentary analysis.

STAGE 1: DEFINE KEY POLICY MILESTONES

Key policy milestones are identifiable through reviewing the heritage of the current policies: what were the key events, perspectives, legislation, and priorities of the past that contributed to any significant change in end-of-life care services and/or policies in a particular location? Alberta has a strong history of palliative care events and directions. Table 1 is the result of a two-stage process: an original rendition of the timeline, based on a documentary analysis, was sent to the key informant prior to the interview. The interviews helped to clarify, confirm, and/or add to the timeline; as a result, changes were made. The timeline is therefore informed by the documentary analysis and elaborated on the key informant interviews.

TABLE 1: *Trajectory of Policy and Related Events Impacting Design and Delivery of Palliative and End-of-Life Care Services in Alberta (based on document analysis and key informant interviews)*

1985
1989: Home Care has one Palliative Care Team in Edmonton

1980
1981: Dr. Helen Hays founds the Palliative Care Unit: 1) one unit at the General Hospital in Edmonton; 2) consult services at Misericordia Hospital (acute care facility located in Edmonton)

1975
1978: Dr. Esther Robins begins the first Canadian CanSurmount program for cancer survivors at Foothills Hospital (Calgary)

1940–1970
First free cancer services program established in Alberta (first in Canada)

1940–1970 – 1975 ——— 1980 ——— 1985 ——⟶

1990: Division in palliative care medicine created at the University of Alberta (Edmonton)

1991: Home Care Regulation: Palliative Care clients exempted from "no provision of 24 hr. continuous service/exemption of palliative clients from monthly service of $3000/mos."

1992 (approx.): Division of Palliative Medicine established at University of Calgary

1993, December: Alberta Health creates "Palliative Care: A Policy Framework" (defining PC service limit; plans for end-of-life services; and core services by all regional health authorities)

1993: Advisory Committee formed for the purpose of designing the Regional Palliative Care Program (Capital Health, 2007, p. 6)

1994: Government of Alberta establishes Provincial Health Ethics Network, which facilitates the ethical examination of individual decision-making related to health and quality of life

1994: Pilgrims Hospice, a new non-profit agency providing end-of-life services (Edmonton), established

1994: Alberta government regionalizes the delivery of health care by creating 17 new geographic entities: regional health authorities

1995: Regional Palliative Care Program in operation (Edmonton), funded by Capital Health

1995: Tertiary Palliative Care Unit opens at Grey Nuns Community Hospital (part of the Regional Palliative Care Program in Edmonton)

1995: Establishment in Edmonton of the Capital Health Regional Program

1999–2001: Pallium Project—Phase I, II and III (Health Canada) aims to improve palliative care in rural western and northern Canada (see Wilson Associates, 2002)

1995–1998: Chinook Health Region Palliative Care Program created

1995–1996: Rural Physician Action initiative established by the Alberta Medical Association to attract physicians to rural settings

1997: Lakeland Palliative Care Project established (funded by Lakeland Regional Health Authority)

1998: First rural palliative and end-of-life care program in Chinook Health Region (rural physician training in palliative care)

1998 (approx.): David Thompson Health Region Palliative Care Program created

1998: Calgary Regional Health Authority establishes the Regional Palliative Care Program

1998: Publication for practitioners (nurses): *99 Common Questions (and Answers) about Palliative Care: A Nurse's Handbook* (Capital Health Authority, 1998; rpt. 2001)

1998: Two rural regional focused palliative care programs exist in Alberta (Chinook Health Region & Capital Health Region)

1999: In Calgary Health Region, four evaluation studies determine family physicians' views of palliative care services (project incl. literature review, focus groups, a priority-setting exercise, interviews, forced-choice and open-ended surveys, and chart audits)

1999: Edmonton Symptom Assessment Scale (ESAS) validated as a reliable instrument for measuring nine symptoms in palliative care patients (Dudgeon, Harlos, & Clinch, 1999)

1999 (approx.): Hospice opens in Lethbridge to serve Lethbridge and Chinook rural communities

1999–2001: First Canadian distance-learning program in palliative care for MDs and RNs, focusing on rural health care providers

1990 ——————— **1995** ———————→

2000

2000: Nurse practitioners introduced in Alberta (15 in 2000)

2000: Alberta government conducts study to improve quality of palliative care for cancer patients (who constitute the majority of palliative care recipients) in the Calgary Health Region

2000: Adoption of a policy to establish a new model: for every palliative patient, there would be 1 home care RN and 1 family MD (AB03, p. 2)

2000–2001: East Central Palliative Care Program (near Camrose)

2001: Alberta Cancer Board publishes *Alberta Hospice Palliative Care Resource Manual* (Alberta Cancer Board, 2001)

2001: Palliative Care Program Council replaces advisory committee

2001, October: Community Care Access becomes community referral link to tertiary care, community consultation, and home care (i.e., all centralized)

2001: Four sites opened for palliative hospices by Capital Health (Edmonton and St. Albert)

2002: Courses established for rural family medicine residents in Alberta

2002 (approx.): New Palliative Care Program in Palliser Health Region (Medicine Hat area)

2000–2002: Alberta funds study to develop a formal referral process at the Tom Baker Cancer Centre to aid in the transition of palliative patients back to home communities

2003 (approx.): Palliative Care Unit opens at Red Deer Regional Hospital

2003: Pilot testing of an online journal club for rural practitioners

2003–2006: Pallium Project Phase III: broadening of palliative care related services and programs in Alberta, Saskatchewan, and Manitoba

2003: Calgary begins development of a rural palliative care team

2003, October: Capital Health/Caritas Health Group Palliative Care Conference explores dying; Conference theme: "Reflections on Dignity in Palliative Care"

2003: Alberta reduces number of regional health authorities to 9; 7 are largely rural; Lakeland Palliative Care Program shuts down as a result (AB05, p. 1)

2003: Establishment of rural family practice residency program

2003: Primary Care Initiative Agreement: Alberta Medical Association, Alberta Health and Wellness, and Alberta's regional health authorities outline a provincial approach and objectives: increase the number of Albertans with ready access to primary care; manage access to round-the-clock primary care; increase emphasis on health promotion, disease and injury prevention, care of patients with complex problems and chronic diseases; improve co-ordination of primary health services; foster a team approach to primary health care (Primary Care Initiative Committee, 2008)

2004, August: Minister of Health and the Province of Alberta remove per diem cost of hospice services

2004–2005: Alberta netCARE Electronic Health Record developed as database of health information; some palliative care information, such as drug coverage, recorded

2004–2005: Development of ASAP (Alberta Strategic Alliance for Palliative Care), bringing together key rural decision-makers to address gaps in services

2000 ⸻⸻⸻⸻⸻⸻⸻⸻⸻⸻⸻⟶

2005

2005: 130 nurse practitioners in rural and remote regions in Alberta

2005: Additional funding provided to primary care networks; palliative care a key focus (ABo3, p .3)

2006, April 27: *Employment Standards (Compassionate Care Leave) Amendment Act* comes into force in BC; compassionate care leave legislation now exists in every Canadian province except Alberta

2006: Alberta introduces Palliative Care Drug Supplement Plan

2006: Palliative Care Units: Edmonton: 1) Palliative Care Program, University of Alberta Hospital; 2) Palliative Care Program, Royal Alexandra Hospital

2006: Palliative Care Initiative implemented; as of September, 18 Primary Care Networks exist, with palliative care as one core service (Primary Care Initiative Committee, 2008)

2006–2007: Alberta government provides $500,000 to improve hospice palliative and end-of-life care: two-year project Helping Operationalize Palliative Expertise (HOPE) focuses on information sharing, standardizing care, and enhancing end-of-life services

2007: Alberta Health and Wellness introduces Continuing Care Health Services Standards; some focus on palliative and end-of-life care (e.g., service co-ordination and quality improvement)

2007: Aim to have standards for Hospice Care in Professional Accreditation Programs for health care practitioners

2007: New Palliative Care Program in David Thompson Health Region (Palliser) with nursing support and physician consultation support at the community level

2005 ⟶

In addition to the key policy and related events are specific accounts by key informants about the overall state of palliative care in the province, as they understand it over time. One key informant, for example, describes the nature and evolution of palliative care services in Alberta in this way:

> palliative care has sort of rolled out in Alberta [it] has been an urban to rural phenomenon where the urban programs have developed and gotten themselves in a position to sort of get the job done and then the rural programs have largely sort of developed or been modelled after that. (AB04, p .1)

Palliative care services in Alberta were also described as being quite centralized previous to 2003, when expertise was centred in the major cities of Edmonton and Calgary. Rural practitioners had to access these services in one of these two urban centres:

> if somebody [e.g., a patient] was complicated out in a rural community...they could get expert care if they got transferred into Edmonton or Calgary...within the tertiary palliative care unit and then got sent back home to their rural communities with a bunch of expert advise and kind of "call us if you need us" sort of thing. (AB04, p. 4–5)

The model said to be used first by Edmonton in 1995, followed by Calgary and then by the Chinook Health Region, was described as an integrated palliative care service model: "when Edmonton's program started taking shape then it was probably the biggest change in the province that allowed other programs [in Calgary and then in Chinook] to step forward" (AB04, p. 3). Although rural practitioners (e.g., family doctors, home care nurses) were said to know how to call on expertise from the urban centres, they lacked the extra support required to provide quality services to those residing and dying in smaller rural communities.

Finally, one other key informant describes the regionalized model of health care used in Alberta as one factor that highly influences palliative care services in general. Although a regionalized model offers a great deal of independence and authority to a region, it was said that this model does not force a region to prioritize any one particular health issue, which may have negative consequences. With a regionalized model, for example, regions are not compelled to take on any particular priority direction: "the environment is such that Alberta Health hasn't said this [palliative care] is something you must do and that you must report back to us and you must meet certain standards, and you must tick off these tick boxes to say that you are doing this" (AB04, p. 13). Because of the shift from a centralized to a regionalized model of providing health care, boundaries between regions have been clearly set, making collaboration between regions quite impossible: "it's hard to go knocking on the next door...and say sure, we will provide services that cross regional boundaries" (AB04, p. 15).

STAGE 2: LOOK AT THE WIDER POLITICAL AND GOVERNANCE CONTEXT

This step in the policy analysis process developed an understanding of the broad social and political trends influencing palliative care services in Alberta. More specifically, it took into account trends specific to change, agents of change, and key factors of resistance in palliative care associated issues, events, and/or policies. At this stage—Stage 2 in Springate-Baginski and Soussan's (2001) policy analysis process—significant policy drivers begin to emerge, as do the obstacles and challenges associated with policy progress in palliative and end-of-life care in Alberta. The following themes evolved from key informant interviews and help to describe the wider social, political, and governance context.

Role of Individual Leaders and Agents of Change (Social Context)

All key informants emphasized that there continues to be strong leadership and influence by key individuals who have made, and continue to make, huge contributions to palliative care services in Alberta. Key informants in this study described these powerful "agents of change" as follows:

> One of the leading persons [a registered nurse] was [name...she/he] was a real mover and really did a remarkable job in getting the program up and running...[he/she] set up a very successful program. (AB05, p .2)

> The person in charge [administrator of a palliative care program/ RN] of setting it up was [name]...[she/he] is a remarkable [person] and very supportive of palliative care. (AB05, p. 2)

[A few registered nurses] were very, very politically active and clinically active. (AB03, p. 8)

Those palliative care nurses (and clinical nurse specialists)...are out
seeing patients doing a lot of work in terms of promoting palliative
care, e.g., education, speaking...[and] all this stuff that happens on
a different level in rural [Alberta]...there may be prominent, well-
known leaders...but you have people working in rural areas that
very clearly are connected to people who are doing fundraising and
service groups...in rural areas you don't live in a clinical world, you
just live out there and as such, you are connected to other service
groups. (AB04, p. 12)

[A certain psychiatrist from outside of Alberta]...had huge char-
isma...a very exciting person...[she/he] sort of started a volunteer
program...[which] permitted [people] to die at home with a team of
volunteers who are highly trained...[she/he] helped to get us really
intrigued. (AB02, p. 2)

[One particular physician] brought in a whole lot of policies and
procedures for palliative care...[she/he] is still very much front and
centre...that has certainly left a huge mark. (AB02, p. 7)

You have to have strong leaders...to push it all forward. (AB01, p. 8)

A number of specific individuals were identified by key informants when
referring to those that moved or drove policy and/or service change in palliative and end-of-life care services. One story was told about the influence
of an individual initiative (change agent) who contributed to advancing palliative care services in Alberta. The creation of Alberta Strategic Alliance for
Palliative Care began in 2005. At that time, one individual brought together
health-related decision-makers associated with rural Alberta to identify
gaps and explore and implement solutions to fill such gaps in order to
improve end-of-life services in the rural areas of Alberta.

Reduction of Regional Health Authorities (Political Context)
In 2003 (effective December 1), the Government of Alberta reduced the
number of regional health authorities from 17 (established in 1994) to 9.

This had both negative and beneficial implications for palliative care services and for related events and projects. One informant described a major negative impact:

> when the Alberta government reduced the number of Regional
> Health Authorities it basically, literally, overnight shut down this
> palliative care program...the nurses were given their pink forms
> within a few days...and it [the Lakeland Palliative Care Program
> of the Pallium Project] was a really remarkable program...the new
> person in charge of the health ministry of that region basically
> said that the palliative care services will not change...they had
> just destroyed...Canada's best example of a successful rural pallia-
> tive care program and service...that was quite a loss in 2003.
> (AB05, p. 1)

Another key informant concurred: "[The Lakeland Health Region]...got chopped into 3 pieces and none of the pieces had enough sort of critical mass to maintain or to continue the palliative care program" (AB04, p. 3). When regionalization occurred, this essential program was lost, and "this kind of flagship rural program suddenly was no more" (AB04, p. 4).

This political action of creating fewer regional health authorities in 2003 had a negative influence in the East Central Region as well. This region was described as having a successful model of palliative care service delivery. However, its boundaries were changed when the provincial government reduced the number of regional health authorities, and so the issue became whether or not rural dwellers would have access to end-of-life care services. After that, palliative care programs in that area "kind of fell apart" (AB04, p. 2). Another key informant agreed, saying that when the geographic boundaries were rearranged, the impact on palliative care services was negative: "[it] chopped up 1–2 rural regions and basically threw a wrench into the works...it added a large rural area around Calgary" (AB04, p. 3).

The rearranging of regional health authority boundaries was in some cases described as having a positive impact on palliative and end-of-life care services. Calgary, for example, because its region now had a large rural component, "had to make very specific steps to develop a rural program... [therefore] it started working on growing and developing a rural palliative care team" (AB04, p. 3–4).

The Value of the Pallium Project (Social and Political Context)

The Pallium Project was implemented to identify rural care and education issues associated with end-of-life care in rural Alberta, Saskatchewan, and Manitoba. The federal government, via Health Canada, committed $4.3 million from 2003 to 2006 to improve palliative care in communities across western Canada and the North (University of Calgary, 2003). A fair number of initiatives were implemented in Alberta as a result of the Pallium Project. Key informants noted that the project had quite positive results for rural palliative care services and programs—all of which occurred as a result of a change of political heart about the value and necessity of end-of-life care services in rural Alberta.

Huge Geographic Distances in Alberta (Social and Political Context)

To create quality palliative care services in rural Alberta, given the province's huge geographic distances, was described by key informants a "daunting task" (AB04, p. 6). For example, there are regions in the north of Alberta that can span 500 kilometres: "there are huge regions and huge areas that it is just extraordinarily difficult to physically travel...[there are] a number of challenges when it comes to different cultures and weather" (AB04, p. 7). The huge distances and the time it takes to travel so far away make the geography of Alberta one of the biggest obstacles to providing progressive palliative care services in the rural areas of the province. The huge distances between locations in Alberta also make it difficult to acquire doctors and palliative care specialists to work in rural communities.

STAGE 3: EXAMINE KEY POLICY ISSUES

Examining key policy issues involves consideration of the relationship between policy issues and livelihood, the main challenges to the pre-existing situation, and the key policy issues used by agents of change to create policy drivers (because such issues are often used as the fuel to generate policy drivers). During stage 3 of the policy analysis process, questions such as how the policy has been responded to and put into action are key. Stage 3 also explores the process used by agents of change to make action happen.

Key informants in this study identified several key policy issues that are driving the need for progress in palliative and end-of-life care in Alberta. Although one key informant (AB03) believed that stronger links are being developed between the home care, primary care, acute care, and long-term care sectors, each independent sector was still highlighted by key informants in Alberta as having unique issues that require distinct policy considerations.

Lack of Rural Focus

As all key informants observed, one of the biggest considerations surrounding palliative care for rural communities in Alberta is the significant lack of focus on rural necessities and special requirements for those needing palliative care services in rural and remote areas. Rural practitioners in Alberta were said to require more support in order to provide quality palliative care services in rural communities. As a result, they develop expertise in rallying that extra support from urban centres to meet existing needs. Williams (1996) discovered similar service inequalities when she explored the development of home care services in Ontario; urban regions are favoured over rural areas.

One key informant talked about the low number of rural palliative care initiatives in Alberta, when referring to a particular point in table 1:

> this rural regional health authority developed its palliative care program in 2001, there needs to be a few more of those...if you do put in all those rural programs that have done some impressive things, its still a fraction of the rural regions in Alberta...there hasn't been the political will in some rural health regions...it [rural palliative care] hasn't been a priority. (AB04, p. 6)

Severely lacking, therefore, are clear policy guidelines regarding priorities for core services related to palliative care, and until now there has been no policy to guide services for rural palliative care.

Home Care Necessities

Several home care considerations exist with regards to promoting policy progress for palliative care in Alberta. Improved end-of-life care supports a model where people, if they wish, can die at home in an environment that is familiar to them and that includes the comfort of family and friends. For this to occur, increased access to home care is required: "there is a huge need...to provide 24 hour a day home-based palliative care services that allow people in rural Alberta to die at home with adequate support" (AB04, p. 14). Currently, sufficient hours of home care are not available to patients (AB06). Because home care does not provide specialized palliative care services, instead providing only "general homecare" (AB04, p. 10), these programs and their practitioners require more specialized education and consultation services. Overall, rural areas in Alberta do not have dedicated palliative home care, as one key informant confirmed: "[home care] often has the greatest needs and greatest demands...because they are at the grass-roots" (AB04, p. 10).

According to another informant, attempts have been made to address home care services as an essential component of palliative care; however, the results have been "mixed...it's some of the rural challenges of the distances traveled [and] the lack of resources" (AB05, p. 7). Home care services for those dying in rural communities in Alberta were also described in this study as being very unpredictable. For example, "when I was doing palliative care 100%, I never knew what to tell families as to how much help they could get from homecare because it would change almost from week to week...it was very unpredictable, I simply had to leave it to families to negotiate with homecare directly because [it] just got foolish" (AB02, p. 6). The pressure on families to negotiate their own care and services was explained as a significant burden (AB02; AB01).

Acute Care Considerations

Because of the weakness in rural palliative care services in Alberta, acute care services, such as small hospitals, provide a lot of end-of-life care services: "there is no hospice-level care in most rural communities" (AB04, p. 10). The result, comments one informant, is a high degree of anxiety on the part of rural hospital staff when someone is dying and at the end of their life. These clinicians are not trained in palliative care and are advocating to the government for educational support.

Long-term Care Influences

Although many individuals live out the end of their lives in long-term care facilities, the approach to palliative care by long-term care staff was said by key informants to be one of "making do" and "getting by" (AB04, 11). One policy issue considered to be significant in the long-term care sector in Alberta, therefore, is the need for a consultation model, which thus far, has not been developed in Alberta in long-term care. Those 65 years and older were said to be driving the need for more and improved palliative care services across the province.

Sharing Expertise: Expanding the Number of Hubs of Excellence

Urban centres have more developed palliative care services than smaller areas in the province. As a result, key informants suggested that these urban centres reach out to support rural communities with consultation and education: "those regions that have a hub of palliative care activity need to reach out to smaller communities...the biggest policy driver...is local support, decentralization, hubs of excellence in the cities...and outreach programs to allow the other [rural] providers to feel supported" (AB04, p. 14).

Overburdened Family Caregivers

One policy driver identified by a couple of the key informants in this study is the huge workload of caregivers looking after dying family members. Not only are they significantly overburdened with the provision of care, but they lack the power to lobby the government for change and support: "they are not always the strongest lobbyists...[and] not able to get together and be powerful" (AB01, p. 5). This lack of lobbying power is likely a result of their overwhelming caregiving role, since it keeps the impact of their role "invisible."

Funding Cuts to Health Services

Cuts to health care funding have been an impetus for palliative care agents of change to respond to various policy-related changes in the field of palliative care in Alberta. Although some palliative care initiatives were said to begin as a result of dedicated funding, limited government money, cuts to home care dollars by the province, and money taken out of hospitals and not transferred to home care, for example, were described as significant reasons for imaginative policy creation and policy change. Such comments as "funding for palliative care has been pulled back" (AB02, p. 8) were common from key informants.

Government Resistance to Change

Key informants identified the provincial government's resistance to change as a significant barrier in influencing change. One story by a key informant describes this further: "then [the] government complained and said they would close us down...eventually government through a lot of local reaction, gave in and said yes" (ABO2, p. 3) and "I don't think there was a lot of political will behind it [palliative care programs]" (ABO3, p. 5).

STAGE 4: UNDERSTANDING THE POLICY DEVELOPMENT PROCESS AND ITS OUTCOMES

Springate-Baginski and Soussan (2001) describe Stage 4 in the policy analysis process as one of identifying and understanding what has already occurred between key actors, regarding policy formulation and the outcomes of actions in terms of the development of broad or macro-level policy. Factors that need to be identified include organizational structures, key actors in the policy development process, strategies to advocate for policy, actors' impact on formal policy-related processes, and the degree of collective action by local groups and/or communities to impact policy (Springate-Baginski and Soussan, 2001, p. 4). This stage looks at macro-level policy in order to understand the local details of what happens to facilitate or deter the policy and policy process.

The level of individual leadership surrounding palliative care in Alberta has been and continues to be very strong. For example, the Alberta Strategic Alliance for Palliative Care is an example of how one change agent collectively brought together palliative care experts to identify service gaps and build solutions to minimize those gaps. As already discussed in Stage 2, many agents of change have played a significant role in influencing end-of-life care-related policies, and these agents have had a significant impact on new directions in palliative and end-of-life care.

STAGE 5: ANALYSIS OF IMPLEMENTATION PROCESS

Stage 5 in the policy process considers the following factors: evidence that the policy produces successes; the level of enthusiasm or resistance to the policy; the pace of policy implementation; changes required to internal procedures and with authorities in government agencies to implement key policies; and an understanding of what had or still has to be done to make changes occur and get people to accept the policies. The successes referred to in this section are based on those accomplishments occurring at the beginning of a variety of palliative care programs, as outlined in table 1. Below are descriptions of some of the outcomes of those successes.

Some Commitment to Palliative Care by Province
and Voluntary Sector Organizations

Although higher levels of political will are still needed, key informants observed that some political support has already existed, to some degree. For example, in the early fall of 2004, the minister of health and the provincial government of Alberta made a decision to eliminate all of the patient's daily costs for hospice care. According to one key informant, this has had a significant impact on palliative care services in the province: "it gave a signal that the government at least was behind the idea that hospice care was something that was sort of as important as other acute care and that it was different than long-term care...and they decided that the care you receive in the dying process should not be a financial burden to people" (AB04, p. 9).

Strong commitment to the promotion of palliative care services by voluntary sector organizations in Alberta is said to be occurring at a grass-roots level. Such volunteer organizations as the Cancer Society and the Alzheimer's Society are demonstrating tremendous dedication, but this is not occurring overtly; it is being provided "quietly" and "in the background" (AB04, p. 9).

Key informants referred to a new movement toward primary care networks in Alberta. The networks are publicly funded and involve family physicians. In a primary care network, a group of family doctors and the local health region work together to co-ordinate health services provided by family doctors, the health region, and other health care professionals. A network may also introduce new programs to provide care for patients, such as a new way to manage chronic illness. Family physicians work with other health care professionals who provide some health services for patients (Primary Care Initiative, 2010a). Primary care networks are a major initiative of the Government of Alberta's Primary Care Initiative, which is an eight-year agreement between Alberta Health and Wellness, the Alberta Medical Association, and Alberta's Regional Health Authorities to advance the way primary care is delivered in the province (Primary Care Initiative, 2010b). Wedel, Grant-Kalischuk, and Patterson (2007) support a definition of primary health care as care that has the ability to transform the way in which the entire health care system functions; it is a model that shifts the focus away from institutional care (e.g., hospitals) and moves the centre of attention to the community level, where illness prevention and health improvement are priority (p. 82). Clearly this supports a change in the culture of health service provision, as outlined in the beginning of this chapter.

One key informant suggested that the establishment of such networks is creating an opportunity to strengthen palliative care services in the province (AB04). This is because one of a number of core services of these networks is palliative care. Some new primary care networks are beginning to explore new collaborations with palliative care experts in order to fulfill the networks requirement to offer end-of-life services; this will strengthen relationships between sectors of health care (AB04).

Continued Need for Political Will and Support

Both the views of the key informants and the documentary analysis demonstrate that some evidence exists that many of the palliative care events and programs aimed at improving services and systems have produced some success. This, however, does not suggest that significant changes are not still required—specifically, the political will on the part of the provincial government.

Major changes are still required to ensure better palliative care services in rural Alberta; the most significant challenge to this, identified consistently by all key informants, is a major lack of political support, will, and direction by the provincial government to strengthen such services. The informants made this very clear: "I haven't seen a lot of political movement in that [palliative care] regard...[there is] minimal recognition from many regional management level structures...it is still not seen as a core service even though it's stated as that...[there is a] lack of political motivation and will" (AB03, p. 5–7). In the words of another informant,

> There hasn't been the political will in some rural health regions...
> it hasn't been a priority. They are too busy putting out other fires...
> there hasn't been a government directive that says that there is a
> minimum standard...that [a] health service must include a palliative
> care service...that probably exists in some document somewhere but
> it hasn't really been enforced. (AB04, p. 6)

For example, the Alberta Strategic Alliance for Palliative Care initiative ended abruptly due to the lack of political support: "the group did not get the kind of support it needed from the Regional Health Authority to...go the next step...[to] influence policy...a group that had a desire to move forward rural palliative care in Alberta but when it came down to funding...actual support from the regional health authorities...[it] didn't fly" (AB04, p. 7).

This same key informant suggests that the result of this overall minimal political support is resulting in health regions acting individually and not collaboratively. With regards to leadership within government, one informant felt that there was no known individual that supported, promoted, or advocated for palliative care services in rural communities: "politically, there have not been any individuals that have stood out in palliative care... [there was not] someone influential on a political level" (AB05, p. 7).

Stories of Success

Having many successful palliative care programs in Alberta has helped to drive, or further influence, more success in this sector; success begets success. Such programs described as being successful were those in Edmonton, Calgary, and Chinook. The Chinook project, in particular, was described by all informants as a model of success: "Chinook...was integrated from the start because their region is largely rural...they have a program that does span the whole region...it's been active for a few years" (AB04, p. 1). It was a program that "went from strength to strength" (AB05, p. 2). The palliative care program in Chinook is made up of a consult team of a handful of physicians and palliative care nurses that provide clinical support in rural areas in the south of Alberta. Currently, this program still continues. East Central Regional Health Authority was also said by some key informants to be a successful example where end-of-life services were well provided in a rural region.

One approach to accessibility has been the use of telehealth, which is beginning to be used in the palliative care sector in Alberta with positive results. A 2006 provincial grant in Alberta to develop rural palliative telehealth programs is providing an opportunity for palliative care experts to offer patient consultation via video. This assists in minimizing the huge geographic gaps between urban and rural centres in Alberta.

From the view of one informant, the palliative care model used in Edmonton played a significant role:

> [It] was really kind of a turning point in Alberta...when Edmonton's program started taking shape then it was probably the biggest change in the province that allowed other programs to step forward...as Edmonton developed their service model in the early 1990s which then Calgary followed then Chinook....Calgary certainly used the work that Edmonton had done in terms of helping to

develop it...to some extent Chinook used the work of Edmonton and Calgary. (AB04, p. 2–3)

Both Edmonton and Calgary, although large urban centres, were deemed by informants to be the gold standard of palliative care because their programs support primary care, offer consultation and education, and are founded on evidence-based research, "and that is what the rest of the province needs" (AB04, p. 16). The Lakeland Health Region was also considered to be a fine model of rural palliative care that was well developed across the entire rural region. It was an example for other communities to look to when creating their rural palliative care services.

The health region surrounding Calgary is highly rural (AB04). A rural palliative care consult team that will go anywhere (e.g., to the home, to acute care settings, to long-term care facilities) to provide consultation for any person at the end of his or her life has recently been created in the Calgary Health Authority. One key informant calls this the "no boundaries approach" (AB04, p. 11) to providing rural palliative care.

There is statistical evidence of positive outcomes as a result of previous and current palliative care initiatives in Alberta. For example, there has been a significant drop in the number of palliative care patients dying in acute care environments (AB05). According to one key informant, after three years of a palliative care program being in place in a particular rural region in Alberta, there was a considerable increase in the number of home deaths: "all of a sudden within one year our percentage of home deaths increased by five times...from 8% to 40%...what it really boiled down to was very proactive surveillance" (AB03, p. 3).

Characteristics of Successful, Rural-focused Palliative Care Services

Key outcomes have resulted from the ongoing development of palliative care service delivery that can be identified as key characteristics of successful rural-focused palliative care services. The following might be seen as some successful benchmarks to explain occurrences that have enabled key palliative and end-of-life programs and policies in Alberta: A strong and ongoing mix of collaboration exists between stakeholders to build program and policy change.

- Palliative care models have an essential and initial link to urban programs before moving outward to rural and remote communities.

- Success brings about further success.
- A health region that includes a large rural component tends to provide rural palliative care services more effectively than a predominantly urban-focused region that has less rural area.
- The greater use of technology, such as telehealth, supports rural service delivery.
- The ability to provide palliative care services to those in varying environments supports a model that includes flexibility, adaptability, and response to changing needs.
- Ongoing commitment (in the form of will and resources) from government is an essential characteristic of rural-focused palliative care services.

STAGE 6: CONSIDERATIONS FOR THE FUTURE—THE LONGER-TERM VIEW

The sixth and final stage in Springate-Baginski and Soussan's (2001) policy analysis process requires an assessment of how current trends affect the future development of policy in order to understand prospects for the future. Key informants involved in this study offered a number of ideas and suggestions for a future of progressive palliative care services in rural Alberta. Direction for the future of rural palliative care in Alberta must consider the exponential growth of the population in Alberta, which will play a significant role in the creation of improved services for those struggling with palliative and end-of-life care issues.

Primary care was identified by several key informants as a sector that has been most responsible for advancing palliative care services in Alberta: "they have been at the forefront of palliative care change in Alberta" (AB05, p. 8). This, however, needs to be supported and enhanced; therefore, direction is needed so that the primary care sector has access to palliative care consultative support (AB03). One of the most recent palliative care programs in Alberta, beginning in 2007 and founded on a primary care model, is located in the David Thompson Health Region in Palliser. This program includes nursing support and physician consultation at the community level. This is a program to keep an eye on, as far as determining the success of primary care in palliative care service provision.

In 2005 and 2006, almost all of the regions south of Edmonton have a palliative and end-of-life care program that offers support, using a consult model (e.g., Calgary, Chinook, Palliser) (AB03). What Alberta now needs, according to one informant, is to offer a secondary or tertiary level of consultation, where the person doesn't have to travel to the nearest urban centre for care. It can be provided right there at the bedside: "that's the place things have to go and they are gradually getting there" (AB04, p. 5).

Some informants emphasized the need to formalize palliative care structures and thus be more stringent in measuring service quality. As one key informant described, some effort is being made in this direction because "we have assumed everybody has access and we have assumed that everybody gets quality care. It has been an assumption that may not necessarily be the case" (AB03, p. 6).

Palliative care initiatives in recent years have been said, by key informants, to demonstrate that the provincial government is supporting, to some degree, ongoing support for improved palliative care services (AB04).

SUMMARY AND CONCLUSIONS

This section provides a synthesis of the palliative care situation in Alberta, as described above, into five major or broad-level themes relevant to palliative and end-of-life care: political, social, economic, cultural, and location of care (see table 2). The need to further synthesize the analyzed data into these themes emerged as a result of our two pilot studies (which took place in Ontario and Prince Edward Island). Such synthesis also serves as a method to promote the integration of the provincial data on policy-related issues in palliative care, framed according to Springate-Baginski and Soussan's (2001) six stages of policy analysis.

The key policy milestones of palliative and end-of-life care programs and policy in Alberta reveal an urban-focused model extended into rural areas; rural palliative care, therefore, is founded on an urban-focused model (sometimes with relevant integrations and adaptations). Further, the shift in 2003 from 17 regional health authorities to 9 was a significant turning point.

The political and government context has been one that includes:

1. *Strong individual leadership*, mainly by registered nurses and physicians working in the field of palliative care in Alberta. Characteristics conductive to successful leadership include being a mover, supportive, politically active, clinically active, promoting palliative care education, connected to many people to support change, charismatic, and knowledgeable of successful policies and procedures.

2. *The decrease of regional health authorities in Alberta* was said to result in a closure of some palliative care programs and a major modification of geographical boundaries for palliative care service delivery. Sometimes, this change in boundaries created regions with large rural areas, forcing a need to develop palliative care programs.

3. *The Pallium Project* resulted in an increase of palliative care programs and greater government focus on palliative care services.

The key policy issues relevant to palliative and end-of-life care in Alberta can be described as a severe lack of rural focus, an underdevelopment of home care services (which lack access, specialized knowledge, predictability, and continuity), a burdened acute care system, and an only "adequate" long-term care system. Policy issues also need to focus on methods and processes of furthering the already existing, yet still young, community-based culture through ongoing political support (e.g., political will, resources).

Events identified as key milestones throughout the history of palliative care in Alberta include a degree of commitment and determination by government and the voluntary sector to advance palliative care policies and programs, a general history of successful palliative care programs over the past 30 years that has helped to enable further success, the use of telehealth to minimize practitioners' long-distance travel to provide consultation and care, and, in some communities, the ability to provide services in a variety of environments.

The overall success in palliative and end-of-life policy development and service delivery in Alberta has been a result of several key factors: available resources at relevant times—for example, "having the right people in the right places at the right time" (AB02, p. 11); access to excellent expertise, such as physicians and nurses with specialized knowledge in palliative care; local leadership that fostered "ground up" development; and the use of a primary care model that supports an integrated model of palliative care.

The greatest successes in innovation in palliative and end-of-life care in Alberta, to our knowledge, are taking place in the Chinook Health Region and in the Lakeland Health Region. Both regions are mainly rural, and both are driven by a community-based, "ground-up" process (Wedel et al., 2007). Chinook, for example, "was the first rural, non-metro [palliative-related care] program" (AB03, p. 1) in Alberta. As a social movement, palliative and end-of-life care has become an area that now receives a high degree of public support because "[people] are beginning to experience home death and the support they receive and the kudos are unbelievable.... [someone stopped me the other day and said] I talked to the Health Minister and said to him 'model everything after palliative care programs in the province and you will be alright'" (AB03, p. 5).

TABLE 2: *Synthesis of Alberta Data into Broad-level Themes*

Major, Broad-level Theme	Synthesis of Policy-Related Issues
Political	• Regionalized model of health service delivery (e.g., in 2003 the province went from 17 to 9 health regions) • The Pallium Project advanced palliative care services in Alberta • The lack of focus on rural service necessities is recognized, as are the special requirements for those needing palliative care services in rural and remote areas • Lack of political will and support for rural palliative care in Alberta
Social	• Strong existing leadership by individuals to advance palliative care services • The Pallium Project advanced palliative care services in Alberta • Successful palliative care programs have helped to drive or further influence more success in this sector • The overburdening of family caregivers operates as a policy driver
Economic	• Statistical evidence of positive results of previous/current palliative care initiatives in rural Alberta
Cultural	• Rural palliative care programs in Alberta are being strongly informed by a local community capacity-building model, resulting in a strong community-based culture in the provision of palliative and end-of-life care service delivery
Location of Care	• The huge distances and travel time make the geography of Alberta one of the biggest obstacles to providing progressive rural palliative care services. This has resulted in difficulty recruiting and retaining doctors and palliative care specialists • The huge geographic distances in the province make the provision of health services difficult • Recognition that those living in rural Alberta have special requirements and different need relative to those in urban centres

AUTHORS' NOTE

This Canadian Institutes of Health Research (CIHR) Interdisciplinary Capacity Enhancement Grant (HOA-80057), titled "Timely Access and Seamless Transitions in Rural Palliative/End-of-Life Care," was funded through the CIHR Institute of Cancer

Research and CIHR Institute of Health Services and Policy Research. Acknowledgement also needs to be awarded to Dr. Mary Lou Kelley and Dr. Judy Lynn Richards.

REFERENCES

Alberta Cancer Board. (2001). Alberta hospice palliative care resource manual. Division of Palliative Care Medicine, University of Alberta. Accessed September 9, 2010, at: http://www.palliative.org/PC/ClinicalInfo/ACB%20PC%20 resource%20manual

Alberta Medical Association. (2005). *Alberta medical history fact sheet*. Edmonton: Alberta Medical Association. Accessed April 14, 2007, at http://www.albertadoc-tors.org/bcm/ama/ama-website.nsf/AllDoc/00707B190EE25FC487256F9D0072C B58/$File/FACT_SHEET.PDF?OpenElement

Canadian Institute for Health Information. (2007). *Health care use at the end of life in Western Canada*. Ottawa, CIHI.

Capital Health. (2007). Regional Palliative Care Program annual report: April 1, 2004–March 31, 2005 and April 1, 2005–March 31, 2006. Accessed September 9, 2010, at http://www.palliative.org/PC/RPCP/Annual%20Report%202004%20 -%20%202006.pdf

Capital Health Authority. (1998). *99 common questions (and answers) about palliative care: A nurse's handbook* (1st ed.). Edmonton: Regional Palliative Care Program, Capital Health Authority.

Dudgeon, D.J., Harlos, M., & Clinch, J.J. (1999). The Edmonton symptom assessment scale (ESAS) as an audit tool. *Journal of Palliative Care, 15(3)*, 14–19.

Field, M.J., & Cassel, K. (Eds.). (1997). *Approaching death: Improving care at the end of life*. Washington, D.C.: National Academy Press.

McKnight, J., Kretzmann, J. (2005). Mapping community capacity. In M. Minkler (Ed.), *Community organizing and community building for health* (pp. 158–72). Piscataway, NJ: Rutgers University Press.

Minkler, M. (2005). *Community Organizing and Community Building for Health*. Piscataway, NJ: Rutgers University Press.

Minkler, M., & Wallerstein, N. (2005). Improving Health through Community Organization and Community Building. In M. Minkler (Ed.), *Community Organizing and Community Building for Health*. Piscataway, NJ: Rutgers University Press.

Northcott, H.C., & Wilson, D.M. (2001). *Dying and death in Canada*. Aurora, ON: Garamond.

Premier's Commission on Future Health Care for Albertans. (1989). *The rainbow report: Our vision for health*. Chair. Lou Hyndman. Edmonton: Government of Alberta.

Primary Care Initiative. (2010a). About PCI. Accessed June 5, 2010, from the Alberta Primary Care Initiative website: http://www.albertapci.ca/AboutPCI/Pages/ default.aspx

————. (2010b). PCI governance and structure. Accessed June 5, 2010, from the Alberta Primary Care Initiative website: http://www.albertapci.ca/AboutPCI/Governance/Pages/default.aspx

Primary Care Initiative Committee. (2008). *Primary care initiative policy manual: Version 10.1.* Edmonton: Primary Care initiative. Accessed June 16, 2010, at http://www.albertapci.ca/Resources/PolicyManual/Documents/PCIPolicyManual.pdf

Provincial Health Ethics Network. Annual report 1999–2000 & business plan 2000–01. Accessed September 9, 2010, at: http://www.phen.ab.ca/society/exec9900.asp

Romanow, R.J. (2002). *Building on values: The future of health care in Canada; Final report of the Commission on the Future of Health Care in Canada.* Ottawa: Queen's Printer.

Sprenger, M. (2005). Issues at the interface of general practice and public health: primary health care and our communities. Accessed September 20, 2007, from the Priory Medical Journals website: http://www.priory.com/fam/gppublic.html

Springate-Baginski, O., & Soussan, J. (2001). *A methodology for policy process analysis: Livelihood-policy relationships in South Asia.* Leeds: United Kingdom Department for International Development.

University of Calgary. (2003, December 4). Multi-million dollar federal funding helps improve quality of life in the face of death for Canadians. Accessed April 4, 2007, at http://www.ucalgary.ca/mp2003/news/dec03/palliative-care.html

Wedel, R., Grant-Kalishuk, R., & Patterson, E. (2007). Turning vision into reality: Successful integration of primary healthcare in Taber, Canada. *Healthcare Policy 3(1):* 80–95.

Williams, A.M. (1996). The development of Ontario's home care program: A critical geographical analysis. *Social Science & Medicine, 42(6),* 937–48.

Wilson Associates Inc. (2002). *The Pallium Project: Palliative care leaders; Profile of major areas of responsibility and related tasks.* Edmonton: The Pallium Project.

APPENDIX A

Key Informant Interview Semi-Structured Interview Questions

1. a) Do you feel this provincial *provisional* flow diagram of policy progress describes the historical evolution of Rural Palliative/End-of-Life Care in _____ (*name province*)?
      i.   Is it thorough and complete?
      ii. Do you feel that there is anything missing, if so, where? (e.g., key events, triggers)
      iii. How should it be different? What is missing? And where?
   b) What do you perceive are the federal and provincial level turning points in this flow diagram? Please explain why?
   c) Can you describe or identify any successes or positive outcomes in Rural Palliative/End-of-Life Care associated with those turning points (*as just discussed*)?

d) In this revised flow diagram (*based on their suggested changes/additions/ subtractions, if any*), what do you perceive are the overall successes / positive results in Rural Palliative/End-of-Life Care along this flow diagram?

e) Again considering this flow diagram and the events you may have added, what do you perceive to be presently or have been the challenges along the time continuum in this flow diagram? Why and were they associated with the turning points we just discussed?

f) Have you observed or experienced key or identifiable social forces (i.e., ideas, changes, groups, organizations, people) that have had a major force or impact in this flow diagram which describes Rural Palliative/End-of-Life Care in this province? *(Interviewer: please record a list)*

    i. And, to what degree has each social force exerted influence?

g) Have you observed or experienced key or identifiable political forces (i.e., ideas, changes, groups, organizations, people who take on institutions) that have had a major force or impact on Rural Palliative/End-of-Life Care in this flow diagram? *(Interviewer: please record a list)*

h) Where has _____ (*please repeat the question for each political force, placing each one on the list into the blank*) had an influence along the flow diagram and how much influence has it exerted on Rural Palliative/End-of-Life Care in this province?

i) I am going to list four other policy-related programs. When I list them can you describe how they may or may not interact with or impact Rural Palliative and End-of-Life Care policies in this province?
  1. Home Care
  2. Acute Care
  3. Long-term care
  4. Primary Care

Policy Drivers

2. The next question concerns policy drivers which are key events, key people, that bring about a change in policy. With that definition in mind, what do you perceive as being the major drivers of the policy that depict or inform our Rural Palliative/End-of-Life Formal Care Provision in this province?

Obstacles/Successes in Policy Related Progress

3. a) In this province, what do you understand to be the main obstacles in policy related progress specific to Rural Palliative/End-of-Life Care? (i.e., both formal and informal)

b) In this province, what do you understand to be key successes in policy related progress specific to Rural Palliative/End-of-Life Care? (i.e., both formal and informal)

Direction for Policies

4. a) Currently, in what direction do you believe the policies regarding Rural Palliative/End-of-Life Care are moving in this province?

   b) Currently, in what direction do you believe programs regarding Rural Palliative/End-of-Life Care are moving in this province?

Key Successes Re: Rural Palliative/End-of-Life Care

5. In this province, what do you understand to be the key overall successes specific to Rural Palliative/End-of-Life Care? (i.e., both formal and informal)

6. In this province, what do you understand to be the overall main obstacles specific to Rural Palliative/End-of-Life Care? (i.e., both formal and informal)

7. a) Are there any other policy or program experts whom you feel we should talk to for this study? *If so can you give me a mailing address so I can send them a letter of information?*

   b) Are there any other people from the community (e.g., from NGOs, researchers/academics, community organizations) whom you feel we should talk to? *If so can you give me a mailing address so I can send them a letter of information?*

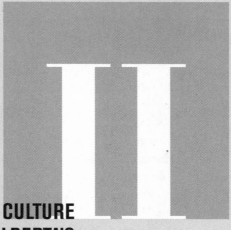

CULTURE
AND ALBERTA'S
INTERNATIONAL
MEDICAL
GRADUATES
(IMGS)

OVERVIEW

International medical graduates (IMGs)—physicians who received their medical degree outside of Canada and the United States—have made long-standing and substantial contributions to health care in Canada. Over the years, approximately 20–30% of Alberta's and Canada's physician workforce have been IMGs.

The four chapters in this section all explore the dynamic interaction between culture and medicine as seen through an IMG-directed lens. We learn of the complexity and richness of the IMG story. The creation of the Alberta International Medical Graduate Program and "mapping diversity" are described. The theme of workforce integration appears in all of these pieces, as do challenges to teacher and learner in the multidimensional, multidirectional process of cultural adaptation.

A personal perspective ("Kamila's Reflection") and a collection of stories arising from a qualitative research project ("Stories of the Journey: International Medical Graduates in Canada") both describe the experience of IMGs. In both of these chapters, the importance of a dream for a better life and the upheaval that follows are illustrated. The very human face of struggle, discouragement, and, for some, success in overcoming barriers is described. We learn from IMGs the importance of connections and supports, and the necessity of cultural adaptation. Advice is provided from IMGs for IMGs who are trying to use their skills as physicians in Canada. The Alberta International Medical Graduate Program, viewed from the perspective of these IMGs, is a "stepping stone" to allow career continuity and eventual medical practice in Alberta.

In "The Merging of Cultures: The Alberta International Medical Graduate Program Experience," the response to an opportunity to better integrate IMGs into the Alberta workforce is described. The program's assessment and orientation activities are depicted, as are program outcomes. The concept of culture in medicine in a Canadian context is briefly explored. Lively physician educator anecdotes complement the program description.

The application of geographical methods helps us understand the "interactions of people and places" in "Mapping Diversity: The Contribution of Geographical Information Systems to the Alberta's International Medical Graduate Program." This chapter includes both mapping and quantitative analysis in response to the question, "What are the characteristics of a successful AIMG Program applicant?" The value of mapping is demonstrated, both as a form of data display and also to help generate questions. The multi-method approaches used here may be useful to others who seek to better understand the complex culture and medicine interface.

All of these chapters celebrate and yet wrestle with diversity. They add to our understanding of the richness of the culture and medicine interface.

KAMILA'S REFLECTION

FOUR

Kamila Saieed MD

I AM ONE OF THE INTERNATIONAL MEDICAL GRADUATES (IMGs) who came to Canada following their dreams of a peaceful life. I am originally from Egypt, where I graduated from medical school in 1986. I worked there for a few years then moved to the Sultanate of Oman, where my husband worked, after I got married. I worked and gained most of my experience there.

My family and I decided to immigrate to Canada in 2001. When we applied we were informed that we'd have to go through an interview. I was told at that time that Canada's demand for physicians wasn't high, and I had to sign a document stating that I would not be able to work as a physician and that I had no right to complain. I went home thinking about it. I always loved my job, and I wondered, "what will I do?" At the end I decided not to think about it and to leave it for the time.

The day came when we had to leave Oman and begin our journey to Canada. I lived in Oman for more than ten years, and it was difficult for me to leave my friends and my patients. It was a very emotional time for me.

Thank you letters, gifts, goodbye parties were thrown to wish me the same success that I had there.

When coming to Canada, we knew that we'd have to start from the beginning. It was so difficult to accept this reality. I started asking people, and I searched the net for jobs that matched my experience. I was told that things were changing for immigrant physicians. At that time I knew about the Alberta International Medical Graduate (AIMG) Program. I started reading about it, and it sounded like an open door that could lead me to continue my career. I decided to challenge the exams, remembering what I was told in the interview and the document that I had signed. I felt discouraged for a while. But at the same time, I felt committed to myself and to my family to challenge the reality we faced at the time. I said to myself, if I had no chance at least I would feel good about trying.

The first year in Canada was the most painful time I had in my life. The culture shock was more than I imagined, and there are no words that could have described my deepest feelings. Homesick, alienated, and "depressed"—or at least that's what my family physician told me. I disagreed with her diagnosis, knowing that I had an adjustment disorder. When times got rough, we questioned why we came. We had everything back home—friends to turn to when in need, families, a house, money, a decent job, a comfortable living. We doubted our reason for immigration. We had thoughts of returning. I started thinking of how I would feel. Defeated? Weak? Or would I feel happy to go back without achieving my goal? After my husband and I debated the situation, we decided to stay for a year and then revaluate our journey.

Doing the Medical Council of Canada Evaluating Examination was the easiest step for me compared to what I faced later. After passing this exam, I decided to go looking for jobs. Everywhere I applied, I was asked the same question: "What Canadian experience do you have?" In one of the interviews, I was asked the same question and I had enough courage that time to tell them, if you give me the chance today then I will gain it, if not I will have none. A week later, I got a phone call from the manager who had interviewed me, informing me that they had a position for me.

My first job in Canada was as a lab assistant in the microbiology department at Calgary Lab Services. When I started working there, I had mixed feelings. I was very happy to have my first job and started making friends at the lab, a very supportive group to work with. But at the same time, when

I remembered my job in Oman and Egypt, and how I was appreciated as a good physician, I cried. I wished I wasn't here.

During my work at the lab, I had finished all the exams required and I applied for the AIMG Program. I was accepted. I left the lab with the wishes of good luck from my friends there, and with a gift: a pen engraved with "Dr. Kamila Saieed," which gave me a push to pursue the dream that I had since day one of arriving in Canada.

I started my residency knowing that my preceptor happened to be the AIMG program director. This made me stressed as I thought, this preceptor, he must have high expectations of IMGs. Language, communication skills, self-confidence, and a different system were but a few problems that faced me. I came from a culture where the patient–physician relationship was a parenting one; the physician would make decisions for the patient, give them a list of "should" and "shouldn't" do's. It was different here. The patient–physician relationship is one of mutual decision-making.

The first problem I faced in my residency was a written complaint from a patient who claimed that I couldn't communicate well with her. This hit me hard. I had a flashback to the time when I used to work in Oman and how I was known to have the best communication skills, always the one to deal with the difficult patients. I said to myself, I'm still the same person, but what has changed? I needed to work on my communication skills to match the Canadian culture.

Most of my experience was with women's issues. In Oman, and most of the Gulf countries, the culture dictated that all women were to go to female doctors and men were to go to male doctors. In the beginning, during my training I wasn't confident or even comfortable dealing with men's issues and that was one of my weaknesses that I needed to work on. The first time I did a rectal examination on a male patient in my preceptor's practice was a challenge. Taking a male sexual history was also initially difficult. With the support of my preceptor, I did learn these skills, in spite of it being very awkward at first.

In the beginning, I found it difficult dealing with patients coming for an abortion. I was born and raised in a culture that always believed that abortion was not an option. It was perceived as killing. If a woman wanted to have an abortion, it was considered an illegal procedure and the doctor performing it would have a bad reputation, and in addition, he or she was subject to licence suspension if someone reported the case. Abortion was something to be done secretly. Moving to a place where abortion was made a right for any woman made me confused. I wondered how I could keep my beliefs without interfering with the care I would give to my patient. Not to judge others was one thing that needed to be clear inside me.

I confess that I felt guilty when I was handling a situation like this. I always wanted to counsel the patient not to go for an abortion, to keep the baby or to give up the baby for adoption. When I did my rural rotation, I had a patient who came from another town because the physician in her town was not dealing with abortion or contraception. He made it a policy in his clinic, and she felt that he was judgemental. At that time I learned the lesson to help my patients as much as I can, not to judge them.

Homosexuality was another difficult issue for me to deal with. Different countries deal differently with homosexuals. In the Middle East they were rejected, dishonoured. It was a shame for any family to have a homosexual member. It was considered something against nature. It was a very embarrassing question for me to ask the patient if he or she had any same-sex relationships, since I wasn't used to asking such questions. It was a matter of time getting used to the culture and the different perspectives that came along with it.

I worked with different preceptors over the two-year period of my family medicine residency program. With feedback from different preceptors, I realized how I had become a different person. "No self-confidence." "Hesitant, but knowledgeable." Those were the comments I initially received. I always underestimated my abilities and I was easily intimidated. I still remember one of the comments from my preceptor that made a big difference: "You need to verbalize your thoughts." I had the knowledge, but I never had enough courage or confidence to speak. I would call this the "IMG tongue-tied syndrome," as I was in contact with some of the other IMGs and they seemed to face the same problems.

I got the chance to work with one of the preceptors who had worked in the Middle East, and he was familiar with the system there. He told me the first day I worked with him that physicians there memorize the facts, but they don't know how to present a case. He was right, but at that time this was not what I needed to hear. I needed to be encouraged and supported. During my times of struggle, some preceptors were supportive while others took pity on me, which in turn worsened my performance. I thought to myself, "How will I make decisions and take care of my patients if I am that hesitant and have no self-confidence?" I was so stressed that I couldn't focus on what I did.

My second year of residency was much better than the first. Rural medicine was my first rotation. I had an outstanding evaluation, which was a driving force for me. I regained my self-confidence. The Simulated Office Oral (SOO) exam was one of the struggles I had. The SOO co-ordinating physician was very supportive. I owe her my success in passing that exam.

At last, I passed my family medicine certification exam. I received my licence and am now qualified to practise as a physician in Canada. I was told this dream would be hard to pursue, and it was one that I always thought would be hard to achieve. But I did it. I'm thankful that I received my training through the AIMG Program. It is a stepping-stone for immigrant physicians to continue their careers in Canada.

THE MERGING OF CULTURES

THE ALBERTA INTERNATIONAL MEDICAL GRADUATE PROGRAM EXPERIENCE

Rodney A. Crutcher
MD, MMedEd, CCFP(EM), FCFP

Peggy Mann BA (Hons)

John Baumber BSc, MSc, PhD, MD

Marianna Hofmeister MA, PhD

Heather Armson MD, MCE, CCFP, FCFP

INTRODUCTION

In this chapter, we explore international medical graduate (IMG) issues from the pragmatic perspective of medical education. We provide a substantive introductory section to set the stage for the Alberta International Medical Graduate (AIMG) Program experience. IMGs seeking to practise in Canada must learn to manage the expectations placed on physicians in the Canadian system. Hence, we address a unidirectional enculturation process. The perspective shared here has been developed from medical education literature and data, as well as reflection on the AIMG Program experience. While there is considerable IMG literature, there is little that attempts to comprehensively integrate the themes we address in this chapter.

To guide the reader, we share some comments here that we hope will be helpful. A comprehensive understanding of our thinking will be achieved by reading the chapter from start to finish. However, some sections have a "stand on their own" quality, so we encourage the reader to read what interests him or her most. To set the stage for the sequential reader, we first make some introductory comments on IMGs in Canada. We then explore our work and the AIMG Program in sections addressing the interplay between medical education and licensure in Canada, and medical education programs overseas. We next address Canadian medical culture and then, arising from this, routes to licensure for IMGs. The AIMG Program is described in the sequence it is experienced by IMGs. We conclude by recognizing and celebrating difference, acknowledging that IMGs' specific knowledge and experience may meet some patient needs ways that a Canadian trained physician's may not. Directions for future research are addressed in the Conclusion to this book.

International Medical Graduates in Canada

IMGs have always made an important contribution to Canada's health care system by supplementing the supply of Canadian-trained physicians. Their presence helps ensure that Canada's physician pool can address the health care needs of its population. An IMG's contribution goes beyond being "just another physician." IMGs help bridge a gap in Canada's multicultural society, bringing new insights into sickness, health, and treatment. They and the Canadian-trained physicians who work with them must bridge cultural gaps in clinical knowledge, skills, and professional behaviours. IMGs must learn to manage the expectations placed on physicians in the Canadian system. Their Canadian teachers and colleagues must learn to work with physicians who bring new perspectives to the practice of medicine.

IMGs are physicians who received their medical degree outside of Canada and the United States. They may be Canadian-born citizens who have gone overseas to study medicine or physicians who obtained their medical degrees in another country before immigrating to Canada. In Canada, the term "IMG" refers to the country in which a physician earned his or her medical degree, not the physician's country of origin. IMGs have consistently represented 20–30% of Canada's physician pool since 1969 (Crutcher, 2002). However, the ease with which they have been able to enter practice in Canada has changed over time. Changes to immigration policies, the medical education system, and provincial regulatory requirements have influenced the number of IMGs entering practice. In the 1980s and through to the mid-1990s, for example, immigration and physician supply policies made it very difficult for internationally trained physicians to become licensed for practice (Crutcher & Dauphinee, 2004).

In the mid-1990s, communities across the country began to experience physician shortages. Many provinces and territories introduced strategies to increase the supply and equitable distribution of physicians in their jurisdictions. Since then we have seen Canadian medical school enrolment increase and the introduction of policies and programs aimed at increasing IMGs' access to licensure (and therefore medical practice). Most jurisdictions now have formalized programs designed to help prepare IMGs for licensure.

The Relationship Between Medical Education and Licensure in Canada

The licensure of physicians in Canada is a provincial/territorial responsibility. Each province and territory has a medical regulatory authority called the College of Physicians and Surgeons. These colleges are the medical profession's elected governing bodies. They are established by provincial or territorial legislation to regulate the practice of medicine (Federation of Medical Regulatory Authorities of Canada, 2007). They do this by ensuring that only physicians who meet established standards in education, qualifications, ethical conduct, professional practice, and continuing competence receive licences to practise medicine. These regulatory colleges also deal with patient complaints and concerns about their physicians.

Provincial licensure requirements can vary; however, certain requirements are common across the country. All physicians in Canada must hold valid medical degrees, have completed a minimum amount of postgraduate medical education, and have passed certain national medical exams in order to practise medicine. In most provinces, the requirements for a full licence include passing the national certification exams held by the College of Family Physicians of Canada (for family physicians) or the Royal College of Physicians and Surgeons of Canada (for specialists), being a Licentiate of the Medical Council of Canada, and being authorized to work in Canada.

The Canadian medical education system is structured so that, in most cases, its graduates are eligible for a full medical licence across the country. The country's undergraduate and postgraduate medical education programs are each accredited by national organizations that set the national standards for medical education.[1] Most people refer to undergraduate medical education programs as "medical school." Medical school involves a mixture of classroom and clinical learning opportunities. The curriculum is designed to enable the acquisition of the basic medical knowledge, skills, and behaviours needed to practise medicine.

Physicians earn their medical degrees once they successfully complete medical school. In Canada, they then enter a postgraduate medical education program or "residency." Residency programs are designed to enable medical school graduates to learn how to practise independently by Canadian standards as a family physician or specialist. Basic Canadian residency programs are two to five years long, depending on the discipline. Medical graduates are considered "residents" during this time. They have gradually increasing responsibilities in providing direct patient care. Residents are under the supervision of a fully licensed physician at all times and may have additional supervision by senior residents. They receive a salary and benefits. Upon completion of a residency program, most residents go on to challenge the certification exams offered by the College of Family Physicians or the Royal College of Physicians and Surgeons of Canada.

Medical Education Programs Overseas

Medical education programs overseas often vary significantly from Canadian programs. There are important differences in educational philosophy, curriculum, learner and program evaluation, and the importance of research. Access to educational, clinical, and technological resources can also vary significantly. Canada enjoys some of the world's most advanced technologies for diagnosis and treatment and a state-of-the-art drug inventory. By comparison, in many developing countries, medical schools and hospitals have limited or no access to basic diagnostic tools such as an X-ray, ultrasound, or electrocardiogram machine. Certain drugs such as "statins" (which lower high-risk cholesterol and triglyceride levels to aid in the prevention of heart disease), "high-end" antibiotics, or chemotherapeutic agents are not available in many countries and therefore "may not exist" from an educational perspective. Why would the interpretation of computerized scans be taught when the student learning or practising in his or her home country will not see one in the foreseeable future?

Various studies have shown that the differences between North American and overseas medical education and health care systems go beyond the scientific basis of medicine. IMGs in American residency programs have noted key differences in the training they received in areas such as mental health, medical interviewing, and patient–physician relationships (Searight & Gafford, 2006). Comparing medical education programs in the United States and India, Singhal and Ramakrishnan (2004) noted that IMGs from India may not have the same exposure to in-hospital training, opportunities to develop physician–patient relationships, or experience with patients of the opposite sex as North American medical students have. Heather Armson, co-author of this chapter, recalls one IMG:

> The international graduate was in her assessment period and had worked with me for one month. She was an excellent physician with good communication skills and an appropriate knowledge base. Near the end of her last week, I asked her what her next rotation would be. She grimaced and stated she would be in obstetrics. I questioned her dismay at this prospect. She stated that obstetrics was all about filling in paperwork. Did she not enjoy delivering babies and caring for pregnant mothers I asked? She reported that in her prior training, her one obstetrical delivery had been an observation with a large group of students, none of whom were allowed contact with the patient. This was her whole experience of obstetrics, except for filling in the prenatal paperwork.

The diversity among international medical education programs reflects deeper differences in the health care systems and cultures in which those programs are based.

Kales et al. (2006) suggest that IMGs may be less likely to diagnose and treat late-life depression, due in part to different cultural attitudes and approaches to depression in the countries in which they were trained. In an Australian study, IMGs indicated a lack of confidence with culturally based medical issues, including medico-legal issues such as privacy and mandatory reporting of sexual abuse (Carlier, Carlier, & Bisset, 2005). These differences may be particularly obvious in approaches to difficult issues such as family violence, sexual identity, medical error, or abortion.

Behaviours with authority figures can also differ significantly in other medical cultures. There may be little emphasis in these programs on self-directed learning, critical appraisal, and evidence-based practice. Many IMGs are accustomed to showing deference to their professors through self-effacement and modesty. They are often not comfortable challenging their teachers and may hesitate to ask questions, as is expected of medical graduates in a North American context as part of their development of problem-solving skills. In Canada, medical graduates and residents are expected to demonstrate certain critical-thinking skills as part of the clinical decision-making process:

Residents in most of the developing countries are supposed to listen and agree with the staff person. No questions can be asked until the end. Silence, agreeing, and moving heads in agreement are considered signs of respect. No independent decision making can be made from the residents part, even simple things like ordering blood work has to be discussed with the staff first [*sic*]...the North American...emphasis on independent decision-making was quite a change. (Sannoufi, 2004)

The skills physicians require and the behaviours expected of them can be heavily influenced by the culture in which they are practising. IMGs who are integrating into practice in a new country may have few personal or professional supports to help them address the many stresses associated with the enculturation process. IMGs integrating into the Canadian health care system must successfully navigate the expectations that are placed on them in the Canadian context.

CANADIAN MEDICAL CULTURE
The Concept of Culture in Medicine
The concept of a "Canadian Medical Culture" is hard to define, especially when considering how it is reflected in and influenced by medical practice. We can begin to understand this culture as "an integrated pattern of learned beliefs and behaviours" that is shared by medical practitioners (Betancourt, 2003). These learned beliefs and behaviours include thoughts, communication styles, ways of interacting, views of roles and relationships, values, practices, and customs.

This understanding of medical culture is rooted in a framework of social constructionism. In social constructionism, knowledge is seen "as a participant in the construction of reality" (Lupton, 1994, p. 11). The behaviours and expectations of individuals and groups are rooted in discourses and social practices with deep and complex histories. Based on this cultural framework, we can begin to understand how physicians' medical knowledge, skills, and behaviours will vary depending on the culture in which they trained and/or practised. As in all cultures, Canadian expectations of their physicians are rooted in Canadian norms and institutions. The way physicians practise medicine in Canada is a product of their collective beliefs and behaviours, which, in turn, are shared and shaped by the society in which they serve. While not all physicians will behave in the same way,

FIGURE 1: *Model of Accountability of the Physician*

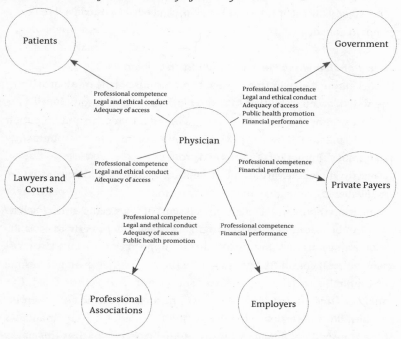

Source: Emanuel and Emanuel, 1996, as modified by Hofmeister, 2007.

the expectations of their behaviours are deeply embedded in Canadian cultural norms.

IMGs in Canada are a diverse group, coming from many different countries. There are often substantial differences in their educational background and clinical practice experience prior to their settlement in Canada. The demographic and educational diversity of IMGs in Canada has been studied in a subset of IMGs who applied to the Canadian Residency Matching Service—the national matching process through which Canadians and, in some provinces, IMGs access residency positions in Canadian medical schools. The majority of IMGs in the study (86.4%) obtained their medical degrees from countries in Asia (central, south, east), Eastern Europe, the Middle East, and Africa (Crutcher, Banner, Szafran, & Watanabe, 2003; Szafran, Crutcher, Banner, & Watanabe, 2005).

While the Canadian public embraces diversity, it also expects all professionals to uphold the standards of care and practice mandated by Canadian professional regulatory authorities. For physicians to assimilate into

Canadian medical culture, they must first acquire and demonstrate the knowledge, skills, attitudes, and behaviours needed to be considered competent in Canada.

Understanding Physician Accountability in Canada

The beliefs and behaviours expected of physicians are the result of an intricate web of accountabilities. In Canada, physicians must comply with the standards set by the regulatory colleges in order to receive and keep their licence to practise. However, physicians must also maintain accountability to a number of other institutions and groups.

Figure 1 shows the various social, political, and economic factors that are core elements of Canadian medical culture today.

The contemporary Canadian expectations of physicians' ethical behaviours can be traced back to the origins of medicine. As early as 1500 BC, Hindu physicians took an oath akin to the Hippocratic Oath taken by physicians today. It committed physicians to the care of their patients, despite any conflicting social norms and customs (Lammers & Verhey, 1998). This patient-centred approach has remained the focus of medicine for centuries. The following version of the Hippocratic Oath, as taken by the graduates of the University of Calgary's Faculty of Medicine, emphasizes this point. The Oath was adopted in 1972 and is based on the modified Hippocratic Oath adopted by the Geneva Convention in 1948:[2]

Oath of Hippocrates

Now being admitted to the profession of medicine, I solemnly pledge to consecrate my life to the service of humanity. I will give respect and gratitude to my deserving teachers and in my turn I will teach and I will study. I will practice medicine with conscience and dignity. The health and life of my patient will be my first consideration. I will hold in confidence all that my patient confides in me.

I will maintain the honor and the noble traditions of the medical profession. I will not permit consideration of race, religion, nationality, ideology, or social standing to intervene between my duty and my patient.

I will maintain the utmost respect for human life. Even under threat, I will not use my knowledge contrary to the laws of humanity.

These promises I make freely and upon my honor.

(Modified Geneva Version)

The contemporary patient-centred approach to health care, which is so central to Canadian medical practice, is rooted in a respect for the individual and an understanding of physicians and patients as partners. Physicians are required to integrate science, ethics, and compassion in their medical practice. Patient care can involve any number of activities, depending on the type of physician and the health care service context. For example, in family medicine, health promotion, disease prevention, and risk reduction are core elements of patient-centred care.

Patient care in Canada is often characterized by the vigorous application of medical science and technology to treat or cure an illness. The application of medical science and technology is guided by the principle of evidence-based medicine. Sackett, Rosenberg, Gray, Haynes, and Richardson (1996) define evidence-based medicine as "the conscientious, explicit, and judicious use of current best evidence in making decisions about the care of individual patients. The practice of evidence-based medicine means integrating individual clinical expertise with the best available external clinical evidence from systematic research."

There has been an explosion of medical research in the past four to five decades. The new information generated by this research has the potential to significantly enhance the health of society and of the individual patient. However, the societal benefits of this research depend on the degree to which physicians translate this new information into their clinical practice. There may be under use, overuse, or misuse of new research information (Sung et al., 2003; McGlynn et al., 2003; Schuster, McGlynn, & Brook, 1998). Despite its potential to positively enhance the health of society, the benefits at the level of the patient can be hampered by a lack of consistent and appropriate application of new knowledge on the part of physicians.

Canadian physicians must address a number of challenges in the delivery of patient care. These include expectations and rules around confidentiality, truth-telling, ethical issues, and informed consent. There are appropriate behaviours that relate to professionalism, resource allocation (balancing the provision of access with prudent use of health care resources), research ethics, and relationships to industries such as pharmaceutics. Physicians must be able to have appropriate conversations with their patients and their families about organ donation, end-of-life decision-making, transplantation issues, abortion, and maternal–fetal dilemmas.

Most physicians in Canada are paid on a fee-for-service basis. They receive itemized payments for patient visits and the procedures they perform.

This has introduced a potential element of expediency into Canadian medical culture. There is an economic incentive in a fee-for-service system for physicians to see as many patients as possible during a day. In recent years, patient volumes in many practices have increased. This is also the result of a shortage of physicians available to meet patients' needs. Physicians will work long hours in order to address the health care needs of their many patients. These factors contribute to brief physician–patient encounters that leave little time to explore less apparent psychosocial issues with the patient. Follow-up appointments may be needed if a patient has more than one health issue they would like to address.

In the last decade, many governments and local/regional health authorities have begun to introduce new, salaried models for primary care physicians. Nurses, nurse practitioners, or allied health care providers such as dieticians or physiotherapists may be integrated into these models, depending on the individual needs of the community. Salaried models take the pressure off physicians to see as many patients as possible in a given day, allowing them to spend more time with a single patient if needed. In turn, the introduction of interdisciplinary teams maximizes the capacity of the various health care providers to meet the range of patient care needs. These new initiatives bring challenges to both Canadian graduates and IMGs who must work to understand and adjust to an interdisciplinary, collaborative approach to patient care. The physician may not be the best leader in complex medical-social issues and must recognize the important contribution of other health care providers with more expertise.

As a result of the proliferation of health-related websites, information about health and medicine has become much more accessible to the average North American. Patients often come to their physician armed with research about the possible causes and treatments for their maladies. They expect that the slightest medical problem will be thoroughly investigated using all the technology available. After all, a headache may be the result of a brain tumour! Physicians must be able to manage their patients' concerns and expectations for treatment within a health care system that rewards thoroughness coupled with an appropriate use of limited resources. Physicians must also mitigate their fear of litigation or a patient complaint to the regulatory college if they "miss" a diagnosis. These conflicting tensions have contributed to the challenges many IMGs face when integrating into Canadian medical practice.

Ensuring the Competence of Canadian Physicians

The Canadian medical education and regulatory systems are designed to ensure that physicians are able to provide safe and effective patient care. The national bodies that accredit the Canadian medical education programs ensure that graduates possess the competencies deemed necessary to meet Canadian standards.

Canadian undergraduate medical education programs are three to four years long, depending on the school. Before entering medical school, most students must first complete a baccalaureate degree. Some students will have completed a master's degree or a PHD prior to medical school entry. The first two years of medical school are largely classroom based, while the third and fourth years are more clinical in nature. During these latter years, medical students do rotations as clinical clerks, where they learn about the different medical disciplines from academic physicians and community preceptors in real-life medical settings.

By the end of medical school students should have developed the requisite knowledge, clinical skills and attitudes for their residency training and subsequent medical practice. Graduates from a Canadian medical school must demonstrate a solid understanding of:

- the professional values, attitudes, behaviours, and ethics of medicine in Canada
- the scientific foundation of medicine
- the communication skills required of Canadian physicians
- the clinical skills required of Canadian physicians
- Canadian population health and health systems
- medical information management structures
- clinical decision-making
- the role of research, critical thinking, and evidence-based medicine (Frank, 2005).

Following medical school, new medical graduates enter a two-to-five year residency program. During this time, the residents are expected to be able to see and treat patients while under supervision. Most rotations within a residency program are preceptor-based. Residents work with a specific physician or team of physicians and their patients. These physicians, acting as preceptors, provide residents with the associated medical education required for that discipline, including supervision and feedback. This system supports the development of core content knowledge coupled with both clinical and critical thinking skills. The goal is to prepare residents for practice in the Canadian context.

The national bodies responsible for accrediting postgraduate medical education programs set the educational standards for residency programs. The College of Family Physicians of Canada's objectives for family medicine residency programs state that "the individual patient should be able to expect a doctor trained as an attentive listener, a careful observer, a sensitive communicator and an effective clinician" (College of Family Physicians of Canada, 1995, p. 4). The objectives align with the "Four Principles of Family Medicine":

- The physician is a skilled clinician.
- Family medicine is a community-based discipline.
- The physician is a resource to a defined practice population.
- The patient–physician relationship is central to the role of family physician. (College of Family Physicians of Canada, 2007)

Similarly, the Royal College has developed a definition of the competencies required for specialist physicians. These are known as the CanMEDS Roles:

- Medical expert (central role)
- Communicator
- Collaborator
- Health advocate
- Manager
- Scholar
- Professional (Frank, 2005).

To fulfill these principles and competencies, the resident must acquire certain knowledge, skills, and behaviours, much of which is learned tacitly and is not always expressly taught. Canadian medical graduates gain their understanding of how to provide safe and effective patient care through experiences in a range of clinical environments. This knowledge is diverse and relates to all aspects of patient care. It incorporates everything from the expected format of patient chart notes to the proper way to present a patient at rounds, to appropriate interactions with nursing and allied health professionals, to the length of the working day.

There are a number of exams and evaluations that residents must undertake before they can enter practice. Residents must pass the Medical Council of Canada's Qualifying Exams Parts I and II. The Medical Council of Canada's examinations assess many aspects of a physician's competence, including patient care and their understanding and application of the Objectives of the Considerations of the Legal, Ethical and Organizational Aspects of the Practice of Medicine (CLEO). Successful completion of these exams, together with at least two years of postgraduate medical education, forms the basis of the Licentiate of the Medical Council of Canada (Medical Council of Canada, n.d.). Once physicians complete their residency programs, they will challenge the College of Family Physicians of Canada or Royal College certification exams. Passing these exams certifies that they are competent to practise medicine according to Canadian standards. Most provinces require physicians to be a Licentiate of the Medical Council of Canada and to have national college certification in order to be licensed.

The College of Family Physicians of Canada and the Royal College play an important role in ensuring physicians' competence once they are in practice. Provincial regulatory colleges require licensed physicians to take a certain amount of continuing medical education accredited by these national colleges to stay current with recent medical advances.

Many physicians also become members of the Canadian Medical Association, which delineates the standards of ethical behaviour expected of Canadian physicians. The Canadian Medical Association serves and unites the physicians of Canada (Canadian Medical Association, n.d.). It is the national advocate, in partnership with the people of Canada, for the highest standards of health and health care. The provincial/territorial arms of the Canadian Medical Association play a leading role in negotiating the fee structures for physician in that jurisdiction.

ROUTES TO LICENSURE FOR IMGS
Provincial Routes to Licensure
IMGs will often meet some but not all of the requirements for a medical licence in a given province. For example, they may have passed the requisite national medical exams but may not have taken a postgraduate medical

education program that is recognized by the applicable national college or provincial regulatory authority. There is no international body that is responsible for comparing or accrediting postgraduate medical education programs in different parts of the world.[3] Countries that wish to determine if an international program is similar to their own must complete their own assessment of its curricula.

The Royal College has assessed a number of international specialty postgraduate medical education programs. To date, the Royal College has identified 29 international jurisdictions that meet the college's criteria for postgraduate medical education (Royal College of Physicians and Surgeons of Canada, 2009). IMGs with medical degrees from one of these jurisdictions are able to apply to the Royal College to have their training assessed. If their training is deemed comparable and acceptable to the Canadian standard, the IMG may challenge the Royal College examination in that specialty. If successful, he or she could go on to obtain a full licence with a provincial regulatory authority, provided the other requirements for licensure are also met.

Some provincial regulatory bodies will grant restricted or provisional licences to IMGs who do not hold national college certification but who have completed a residency program comparable to what they would have received in Canada. In Alberta, physicians in this context (including IMGs) may be placed on the Special Register of the College of Physicians and Surgeons of Alberta. Physicians on this register are permitted to practise under supervision or other specified conditions such as a limited scope of practice. In 2006, 763 of the 6,627 physicians in Alberta (11.5%) were licensed on the Special Register.

Each province has developed its own processes for facilitating the licensure of IMGs who cannot obtain a licence through these available routes. In most cases, IMG programs have focused on assessing IMGs' readiness to enter a postgraduate medical education (residency) program at a Canadian medical school. Many provinces now fund a certain number of residency positions for IMGs. Some provinces also offer practice-ready assessment programs in which IMGs are assessed in a clinical setting for a period of time before a decision is made to give them a full licence to practise medicine independently. In Alberta, IMGs that are not eligible for registration with the College of Physicians and Surgeons of Alberta must apply for one of the dedicated residency positions available through the Alberta International Medical Graduate Program.

THE ALBERTA INTERNATIONAL MEDICAL GRADUATE PROGRAM

The Alberta International Medical Graduate (AIMG) Program is an initiative to prepare IMGs for licensure in Alberta. Created by the Government of Alberta in 2001, the AIMG Program's mandate is to increase the number of international medical graduates practising medicine in the province by providing qualified IMGs with access to postgraduate medical education opportunities in high-need specialties. With many communities across the province experiencing difficulties recruiting and retaining physicians, the AIMG Program provides one way of utilizing the valuable skills of IMGs to help address the health care needs of Alberta's population.

It is estimated that there are over 500 IMGs residing in Alberta who do not meet the provincial requirements for licensure.[4] The AIMG Program runs a competitive, merit-based assessment and orientation service that gives these IMGs the opportunity to access dedicated residency positions in one of the province's two medical schools. As of 2006, the AIMG Program had received 395 applications from IMGs who earned their medical degrees in 55 different countries. The AIMG Program's assessment process determines whether IMGs possess the knowledge, skills, and behaviours they need to function at the level of a Canadian medical graduate in Alberta's health care and medical education systems. Residency training programs select IMGs based on the results of this assessment.

ASSESSING AND ORIENTING IMGS THROUGH THE AIMG PROGRAM

The AIMG Program has grown significantly since its inception. It began in 2001 by offering IMGs access to 11 family medicine residency positions. In 2007 there were 50 entry-level residency positions in 10 different medical disciplines available to qualified IMGs. Figure 2 shows how the AIMG Program has grown over time.

The AIMG Program's assessment and orientation process determines whether IMGs have the knowledge, skills, and behaviours they need to succeed in residency training. As shown in figure 3, there are four main stages in the AIMG Program's process for assessing and orienting IMGs.

Stage 1: Determining Eligibility

The AIMG Program's application process is designed to identify IMGs who meet the basic requirements to enter an Albertan residency program. As part of their application, IMGs must demonstrate that they hold a valid medical degree, meet the program's language proficiency requirements,

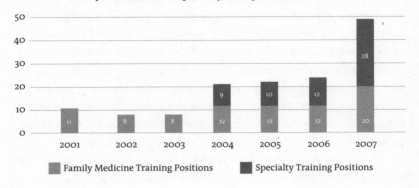

FIGURE 2: *Distribution of* AIMG *Program Residency Positions Across Family Medicine and Specialty Disciplines, 2001–2007*

Family Medicine Training Positions ■ ■ Specialty Training Positions

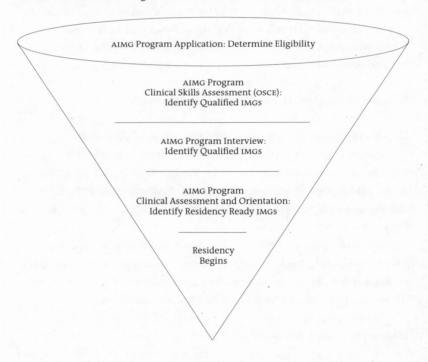

FIGURE 3: *The* AIMG *Program's Assessment and Orientation Process*

AIMG Program Application: Determine Eligibility

AIMG Program
Clinical Skills Assessment (OSCE):
Identify Qualified IMGs

AIMG Program Interview:
Identify Qualified IMGs

AIMG Program
Clinical Assessment and Orientation:
Identify Residency Ready IMGs

Residency
Begins

have passed the requisite standardized national medical exams, and are Canadian citizens or permanent residents. These entry requirements align with the requirements of Alberta's postgraduate medical education programs and the registration requirements of the College of Physicians and Surgeons of Alberta for Canadian graduates. They ensure that IMGs who proceed through the AIMG Program meet the basic requirement for licensure once they are ready for practice.[5]

The AIMG Program's application process assesses IMGs' credentials only. Their behaviours are not factored into their eligibility for the program and AIMG Program staff will not meet with individual IMGs during the application process. However, the application process can still reveal a range of behaviours that are inappropriate by Canadian standards. Rod Crutcher, co-author of this chapter, describes his experience:

> Dealing with gifts offered during or after admissions decision-making can be a delicate matter. Gifts during the admissions process are inappropriate and, while infrequent, are occasionally offered by some program applicants who believe it is the proper— or desirable—thing to do. They know that in Canada bribes are not acceptable, but that flies in the face of some of their experience in other cultures where "tips" or "tokens" appear to be the only certain way to achieve a particular end.

> Some cards or simple gifts (i.e., a box of chocolates or some fruit) have been offered as a simple "thank you" after the conclusion of the admissions cycle. Such gifts have been graciously accepted and shared by our AIMG Program staff in the same spirit in which they were given. Yet even this can quickly become tricky. The limits of the acceptable can be pushed and all assessment programs need to have well defined boundaries.

> I have been offered clothing—an ornate belt comes to mind that was, apparently, hand crafted for me in a far away place. I will never know if the size was correct! Invitations to lunches or evening events can be offered to program staff. A "no thanks" becomes easier after realizing that sometimes the gifts or offers do have "strings" attached and can put the program in a compromised position.

> Equity, rigour, and optics are important in selection decision-making. There is a need for some humour and understanding—and some humility at how this can all play out—notwithstanding

program or institutional policy. At a meeting of program director colleagues, we discussed the boundaries of gift giving and receiving in a cross-cultural setting. A program director colleague smiled and informed me that some time ago a candidate was very insistent and desirous of program entry. My colleague was asked to do all she could, and was offered a pink Cadillac if a residency training position for this individual could be created.

Stage 2: Identifying Qualified IMGs

Not every IMG with the required credentials is qualified to enter a residency program in Alberta. The second stage of the AIMG Program's assessment process helps determine if eligible IMGs possess the knowledge, skills, and behaviours they need to succeed in residency. The program uses an Objective Structured Clinical Exam (OSCE) and a formal interview process to identify qualified IMGs.

The OSCE: The OSCE is a widely used examination format in which candidates rotate through a series of stations where they are required to perform a clinical task (or tasks) with a standardized patient.[6] The AIMG Program uses the OSCE to assess and measure IMGs' clinical skills, communication skills, and language proficiency as compared to a Canadian medical graduate. Standardized patients, who are either people trained to portray a patient scenario or actual patients using their own history and physical exam findings, are used to mimic real-life situations in a series of OSCE stations. In 2006, IMGs participating in the OSCE were asked to complete ten stations and two written tasks, taking ten minutes for each. The stations assess IMGs' understanding of the elements of medicine taught in Canadian medical schools, including their:

- ability to obtain a relevant history and perform a focused physical examination
- ability to outline diagnostic impressions and ongoing management
- interpretation of laboratory results and X-rays
- communication skills
- counselling skills
- ethical issues
- English language proficiency.

Clinical examiners completed a standardized checklist on the IMGs' performance at each OSCE station. These results were collapsed into three categories: clinical scores (weighted at 70%), communication skills (weighted at 15%), and language proficiency and written English (weighted at 15%). Candidates whose OSCE scores were above the minimum acceptable score are considered for interviews.

OSCES are a valuable form of assessment. Much like the simulators used to teach pilots to fly before using real planes, OSCES provide safe, real-life situations for the assessment of IMGs' clinical skills. The OSCE can prove challenging for many IMGs, however. The knowledge and skills assessed and the format and content of the evaluation process may be significantly different from anything IMGs have experienced before. Many IMGs are used to paper and pencil tests as a way of evaluating knowledge. OSCES, in contrast, assess IMGs' ability to assess scenarios critically and perform clinical tasks. By placing IMGs in a simulated environment, OSCES create a situation in which IMGs can be evaluated on the process and outcome of the task.

The Interview: The vast majority of North American medical schools use interviews to predict which candidates are likely to succeed in their programs. While interviews are conducted in different ways, most pose questions to potential candidates about their past or future behaviours. An IMG's performance during an interview provides a sample of the interpersonal behaviours he or she will bring to a residency program. During the interview, IMGs must draw on their English language proficiency, communication skills, and cultural knowledge to respond to carefully generated questions. Through the IMG's responses, interviewers can assess if the person possesses certain attributes required of medical residents, such as integrity, professionalism, and teamwork.

The AIMG Program uses both the OSCE and formalized interviews in its assessment process because each tool addresses different things. IMGs who score very well on the clinical skills assessment may do very poorly in an interview. Rod Crutcher describes one applicant's experience:

> After all the program entry decision-making was over for that application cycle, she asked to meet with me. She wanted to learn what she could do to become a stronger applicant the following year. In

preparation for this, I reviewed her file once more. Yes, the paper-work was fine—exceptionally good, actually. She had performed very well on our OSCE. But the scores from her interviews were poor and the interviewers' handwritten comments indicated a perform-ance that was, at best, mediocre. This surprised me as her referees and others had attested to her excellent interpersonal skills.

We talked and tried to sort out what had gone on. In our con-versation it was apparent that she was articulate, personable, and insightful. It surprised me her interviews had gone badly, and I told her as much.

I asked, "What was the interview process like for you?" I was told, "I thought it went OK. I did what I was taught to do when being interviewed. When I was asked questions, to show respect, I looked down and tried to say as little as possible. I crossed my hands together in my lap and was polite. It was difficult to say anything about myself—in my culture, you would never do that. I would just show my file."

This story reflects how what is considered "appropriate" behaviour in an admissions interview is subject to cultural interpretation. The interviews conducted in the AIMG Program implicitly measure the tacit knowledge, skills, and behaviours expected of residents in an Albertan postgraduate medical education program. The story above exemplifies how respect can be shown differently in different cultures. As constructivism points out, cultural knowledge constructs reality. Behaviours that do not meet the interviewer's expectations may leave the impression that the individual does not have the desired trait and, as such, may not be deemed competent in the North American context.

For the first six years, the AIMG Program used a behavioural-descriptive panel interview for the family medicine interviews, while specialty pro-grams conducted their own in-person interviews with IMGs. Each family medicine applicant was interviewed twice by a pair of interviewers, and each interview was 45 minutes long.

Research into the behaviourally based interview formats indicated a high degree of variability among interviewers' scores for the same performance. Responding to this, in 2006 the AIMG Program piloted a new interview format—the Multiple Mini Interview—for its family medicine candidates.

The Multiple Mini Interview's multi-sampling technique generated stable scores for the traits evaluated, making it a more reliable assessment tool for the program. Comments made by IMG applicants on a post-interview survey indicated that, while the interview was still challenging, they accepted the new format and appreciated the change from the previous one. As one applicant remarked, "There is no way to prepare. You are how you are. Show where you stand."

Stage 3: Identifying Residency-Ready IMGs

Residency program directors use the results of the OSCE and the interviews to rank IMGs for entry into the four-month clinical assessment and orientation phase. This four-month period is the final step before IMGs are selected for a residency program. The AIMG Program shares responsibility with residency training programs for this four-month period. The AIMG Program provides the bulk of the orientation while the residency training programs provide the bulk of the assessment. The clinical assessment and orientation phase is structured much like a residency program in that IMGs interact with patients in real-life settings while being supervised and assessed by physician preceptors. Physician preceptors have a unique role during this time. They support IMGs through the process of enculturation while also assessing their readiness to enter residency.

Depending on their backgrounds, IMGs may not have had the opportunity to pick up the tacit knowledge, skills, and behaviours expected of Canadian physicians to the same extent as Canadian medical graduates. IMGs' lack of tacit knowledge about how to function successfully in a residency program can have a number of direct and indirect impacts on the learning environment. Some IMGs have commented on the differences:

I never heard of SOAP [subjective, objective, assessment, plan] notes until this program.

Documentation is a huge issue here. Not just documenting in a professional way, but in a legal way. Every word is important.

I don't know how to interact with other staff in the office, like nursing staff. In India, they would never question a doctor...also it is hard to figure out who does what here.

Canadian preceptors working with IMGs may interpret a lack of understanding about how things work as a lack of motivation or interest in the issue being discussed. IMGs may also have unrealistic expectations of the clinical assessment process. The result can be limited teaching or a tense learning environment, as Rod Crutcher's experience demonstrates:

I had worked with this internationally trained physician for about eight months. She had practiced in the Middle East and had come to Canada for additional training. She adapted reasonably well to my family medicine teaching practice setting. Her knowledge base was solid, and she had a foundation of good clinical skills. She was willing to learn. She did have some challenges in relating to some of my male patients. Additionally, as with many other residents I have worked with, she had some difficulties competently and efficiently addressing the concerns of patients who presented with multiple medical issues. Time management was an issue.

I had given her periodic, constructive, behaviourally based verbal feedback during the rotation. At the end of the two-month family medicine block, we met for a scheduled performance review as part of completing the final rotation resident evaluation. I recognized that this resident had strengths but still some obvious learning to do.

On our performance review form a Final Rating box had to be checked, with the available ratings ranging from Failure to Superior. Compared to the many other residents I had rated and, given our program standards, I found her overall performance to be mid-level. I checked the "Average" box.

I reviewed and discussed the documentation I had completed along with the feedback shared by others with the resident at our meeting. When she saw her "average" rating she exploded with rage. "I have never been average in my life, and I am not going to be average now. I've always been told I am exceptionally bright and accomplished—I will not be average."

My attempts to explain how I came to this decision and how our rating scale worked was of no comfort to someone who viewed herself and seemingly had been viewed by some others as "the best of the best." She had difficulty accepting that the expectations placed on physicians in the Canadian context may be different than in her previous experiences. Our working relationship was strained for some time. Learning about the "culture of assessment" was difficult for both of us.

The AIMG Program helps to bridge the cultural gap that many IMGs face by providing them with a formal orientation on Alberta's health care and medical education systems during the four-month period. The program offers a series of biweekly sessions that address various cultural, stylistic, and business aspects of medicine. The core content of the sessions covers issues such as professionalism, patient-centred care, evidence-based medicine, use of community resources including allied health professionals, and the medical/legal aspects of medicine in Canada. Session topics have included such things as:

- Professionalism, ethics, and medical/legal issues
- Approaches to teaching and learning
- Patient-centred care, evidence-based medicine, and clinical practice guidelines
- Community resources and the role of allied health professionals
- Provision of health care to specific populations (e.g., Aboriginal, immigrant groups)
- Palliative care and the continuing care system
- Pharmacy
- Library sciences.

These biweekly sessions give IMGs the opportunity to integrate what they learn into their clinical experiences.

The opportunity for IMGs to reconnect with their peer group is also a valuable part of these sessions. Every two weeks, IMGs have the chance to debrief and decompress with their peers. In 2007, the AIMG Program also introduced a mentorship component that partnered IMGs in the clinical assessment and orientation program with AIMG graduates. This mentorship program was designed to give IMGs the opportunity to ask questions and advice from people who had "been there."

Recognizing that all parties must be involved in efforts to bridge the cultural gap, the AIMG Program also offers faculty development and information resources to support physician preceptors in their work with IMGs. These resources set clear learning and evaluation objectives for the clinical assessment and orientation period. Preceptors and IMGs are encouraged to meet one-on-one at the beginning of each rotation to clarify roles, responsibilities, and expectations. IMGs are encouraged to ask questions and speak up about things they may not know. This dialogue can reduce the risk that behaviours will be misinterpreted and can help create a positive learning and assessment environment.

At the conclusion of the four-month clinical assessment and orientation period, residency programs make a final determination of an IMG's readiness to transition into residency. At this point, IMGs leave the AIMG Program and begin the next stage on their path to licensure.

Residency Training

As of October 2007, 142 IMGs had accessed a residency position through the AIMG Program, of whom 49 had completed their programs and entered practice; the rest were still in training. While most IMGs selected through the AIMG Program function well in residency, some need additional time or support. A review of AIMG Program data (2001–2006) reveals that of the 94 IMGs who had accessed a residency position through the program by 2006, 12 (13%) had, at some point in their training, either been placed on probation or were identified as requiring additional training (remediation) prior to rotation or program completion. Figure 4 shows the percentage of IMGs that have needed this support to date. The most common reasons for requiring probation or remediation include a lack of appropriate knowledge for the level of training, gaps in communication and clinical skills, a lack of technical and procedural skills, concerns with computer skills, and a lack of confidence in acute care situations.

We do not have comparative data for Canadian medical graduates who have needed additional support in residency. Educators involved with the AIMG Program and family medicine residency training programs have felt that "13% seems low" when discussing probation and remediation rates. There is no information about the duration of the required remediation or the emotional impact of remediation efforts on the learner or teacher.

While IMG residents can have challenges during residency, many IMG residents can also enrich the learning environment. Co-author Heather Armson observes:

A very complex patient with multiple unusual diagnoses was
seen for a new complaint. The presentation was consistent with

FIGURE 4: *IMGs Placed on Probation or Requiring Remediation After Accessing a Residency Position Through the AIMG Program (2001–2006)*

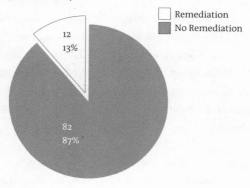

Remediation
No Remediation

12
13%

82
87%

soft tissue tuberculosis but neither the resident nor I had seen the disease except in textbooks. Fortunately, an AIMG resident experienced with a broader range of infectious diseases from his previous training was also working at the clinic. We asked him for a "consultation." He examined the patient, discussed the typical findings and suggested a preliminary management plan. This diagnosis, uncommon in the Canadian setting, was something he had seen repeatedly. He was able to teach the resident and me about the presentation while also reassuring the patient about the typical course of the illness. The patient would have received care within a few days without his input. However, in the referral setting neither the resident nor I would have had an education about the disease and the physical findings associated with it.

RECOGNIZING AND CELEBRATING DIFFERENCE

Much of the literature discussing IMGs has focused on their deficits in medical knowledge and clinical skill (Kales et al., 2006; Kidd & Zulman, 1994; Conn, 1986; Conn & Cody, 1989; Kvern, 2001; Peitzman, McKinley, Curtis, Burdick, & Whelan, 2000). This perspective appears to assume that North American medical schools provide exemplary training superior in all respects to that offered to the IMGs in their country of training. The deficit perspective focuses on what IMGs do *not* know rather than what they *do* know. In contrast, a recent study looking at patient care outcomes revealed no difference in the level of care provided by IMGs and Canadian medical graduates (Ko, Austin, Chan, & Tu, 2005). In some cases, an IMG's specific knowledge and experience may meet patient needs in ways a Canadian physician's cannot.

There are many positive results of integrating IMGs into the health care system. Typically, IMGs are older and have both maturity and life experience. They bring a wealth of understanding of "sickness" and "illness" from their own cultures that can resonate with patients who share similar backgrounds. IMGs provide a window into their respective cultures that may be advantageous given the multicultural nature of the Canadian population. Rod Crutcher observes:

> I have not had to treat many patients with malaria in my Family Medicine practice in Alberta. The closest I usually get to treating malaria is providing travel advice to patients about how to avoid getting it should they be travelling to some malaria-infested part of the world. However, about three years ago, one of my patients came back from overseas and was ill.
>
> My patient had returned from work in a jungle area in Guyana. She had had malaria in the past and suspected she had a recurrence. She had some of the classical symptoms, including sweats, severe headaches, and fever. When I assessed her in the office it was clear that she was quite ill—in huge contrast to her normally robust self. She was dehydrated and hospitalization was warranted.
>
> She was admitted to the local hospital under my care. We started intravenous fluid replacement while investigation was underway. I arranged a consultation with an infectious disease specialist. Over the next day or so, the diagnosis became clear—the patient did indeed have malaria, and a rather severe form of it at that. A treatment protocol was recommended and was started. The specialist requested that I continue to provide care—he felt he would not need to see her again unless there was deterioration in her clinical status. I agreed to the plan, although I was not particularly confident in my own abilities to provide optimal care under the circumstances.
>
> I was on call the following weekend. I had a first-year family medicine resident working with me—an IMG who had trained and worked in Southeast Asia prior to coming to Canada. On Saturday morning rounds, we examined the patient, who looked somewhat

improved and said she felt a little better. However, we noted that she had become significantly anemic ("low blood iron") over the last two days.

My resident and I discussed the matter. I wondered if at some point a blood transfusion might be needed, given the significant drop in hemoglobin? My resident smiled and said to me that prior to coming to Canada she had treated many patients with malaria. She told me that it was not uncommon for them to become anemic. She suggested that no further investigation was needed and that she saw no need at this point for a follow-up infectious disease consultation. She told me that with the present treatment, and a little time, the anemia would be resolved.

Our patient found my resident's calm and knowledgeable reassurance helpful—as did I! And yes, over the next few days, the patient did improve. I thanked my resident for both teaching me and making an invaluable contributing to the patient's care. As physicians we always have more to learn. My IMG resident was an excellent teacher.

Helping to Bridge the Gap

In 2003, the Canadian Task Force on Licensure of International Medical Graduates commissioned a report on the challenges faced by clinical teachers in working with IMGs. This resulted in Health Canada issuing funding for the the Faculty Development Program for Teachers of International Medical Graduates under the direction of Yvonne Steinert and Allyn Walsh. Their report was completed in May 2006 (Steinert & Walsh, 2006).

The Faculty Development Program for Teachers of IMGs addresses six main aspects of working with IMGs:

- assessing learner needs and designing individually tailored programs
- delivering effective feedback
- promoting patient-centred care and effective communication with patients
- untangling the web of clinical skills assessment
- orienting teachers and IMGs
- educating for cultural awareness.

Although the program targets faculty developers, the authors organized the material so that teachers without access to formal group programs can still use it for independent study. In addition to key concepts and teaching and learning strategies, the program includes a variety of web-based teaching tools and resources, including narratives, video scenarios, PowerPoint presentations, and teaching aids, available online at the time of printing (Steinert & Walsh, 2006).

SUMMARY AND CONCLUSION

The concept of a Canadian medical culture, with its integrated pattern of learned beliefs and behaviours, is hard to define and cannot be explicitly taught. While some differences between the practice of medicine in Canada and that in other countries are distinct, many more are subtle and tacit in nature. IMGs wishing to integrate into our medical system must possess the required medical knowledge and be able to function in way that meets the expectation of the public, their patients, and their peers. In turn, their Canadian teachers and colleagues must learn to work with physicians who bring new perspectives and insights to the practice of medicine.

The AIMG Program, in conjunction with IMG programs in other jurisdictions, is part of the Canadian response to the challenge of providing physicians able to provide timely and culturally competent care for our population. It is one example of a structured approach to determine if IMGs possess the knowledge, skills, and behaviours they need to function at the level of a Canadian medical graduate. The AIMG Program will continue to develop its tools and processes to assess IMGs and to help both IMGs and physician preceptors bridge cultural gaps.

The contribution of IMGs to medicine in Alberta and across our country is enormous. We anticipate that these contributions will be sustained into the foreseeable future.

Disclaimer: The views above are those of the authors and do not necessarily reflect the view of Alberta Health and Wellness or the Alberta International Medical Graduate Program.

NOTES

1. Undergraduate programs are accredited by the Committee on the Accreditation of Canadian Medical Schools, while postgraduate programs are

accredited by the College of Family Physicians of Canada or the Royal College of Physicians and Surgeons of Canada.

2. The Hippocratic Oath was modernized in the twentieth century in response to advances in medical knowledge and technology, and the violations of Nazi German physicians during World War II. The modernized version of the oath was adopted by the Geneva Convention in 1948. The University of Calgary adopted a slightly modified version of this oath in 1972 and has administered it to its graduating medical students since this time.

3. The World Health Organization's Department for Human Resources for Health has a World Directory of Medical Schools that provides information on health training institutions worldwide. However, the World Health Organization (WHO) has no authority to grant any form of recognition or accreditation to schools of medicine or other training institutions. Such a procedure remains the exclusive prerogative of the national government concerned (see WHO, 2007).

4. Based on the membership of the Alberta International Medical Graduate Association (AIMGA), as quoted through consultation with an AIMGA representative in the fall of 2006.

5. The AIMG Program also requires IMGs to be residents of Alberta. By assessing IMGs who are already residents of Alberta, the AIMG Program can help ensure that IMGs who obtain a residency position will stay in the province after they graduate.

6. "An SP [standardized patient] is a person trained to portray a patient scenario, or an actual patient using their own history and physical exam findings, for the instruction, assessment, or practice of communication and/or examining skills of a health care provider. In the health and medical sciences, SPs are used to provide a safe and supportive environment conducive for learning or for standardized assessment" (Gliva-McConvey, 2009).

REFERENCES

Betancourt, J. (2003). Cross-cultural medical education: Conceptual approaches and frameworks for evaluation. *Academic Medicine, 78 (6)*, 560–69.

Canadian Medical Association. (n.d.). Mission statement. Accessed September 28, 2008, at http://www.cma.ca/index.cfm/ci_id/44413/la_id/1.htm

Carlier, N., Carlier, M., & Bisset, G. (2005). Orientation of IMGs: A rural evaluation. *Australian Family Physician, 34(6)*, 485–87.

College of Family Physicians of Canada. (1995). *The postgraduate family medicine curriculum: An integrated approach*. Mississauga, ON: College of Family Physicians of Canada.

———. (2007). Four principles of family medicine. Accessed September 28, 2008, at http://www.cfpc.ca/English/cfpc/about%20us/principles/default.asp?s=1

Conn, H.L. (1986). Assessing the clinical skills of foreign medical graduates. *Journal of Medical Education, 61(11)*, 863–71.

Conn, H.L., & Cody, R.P. (1989). Results of the second Clinical Skills Assessment examination of the ECFMG. *Academic Medicine, 64(8)*, 448–53.

Crutcher, R. (Ed.) (2002). *International medical graduate national symposium conference proceedings.* Calgary, AB: Health Canada.

Crutcher, R., Banner, S., Szafran, O., & Watanabe, M. (2003). Characteristics of international medical graduates who applied to the CARMS 2002 match. *Canadian Medical Association Journal, 168(9)*, 1119–23.

Crutcher, R., & Dauphinee, D. (2004, February). Report of the Canadian Task Force on Licensure of International Medical Graduates. Ottawa: Health Canada. Accessed June 5, 2010, from the Canadian Information Centre for International Medical Graduates website: http://www.img-canada.ca/en/pdf/img3.pdf

Emmanuel, E.J., & Emanuel, L.L. (1996). What is accountability in health care? *Annals of Internal Medicine, 124(2)*, 229–39.

Federation of Medical Regulatory Authorities of Canada. (2007). Constitution and by-laws of the FMRAC (As amended and approved by members on June 11, 2007). Accessed September 28, 2008, at http://www.fmrac.ca/about-us/bylaws.html#hpurpose

Frank, J.R. (Ed). (2005). *The CanMEDs 2005 physician competency framework: Better standards, better physicians, better care.* Ottawa: Royal College of Physicians and Surgeons of Canada.

Gliva-McConvey, Gayle. (2009). Definition of an SP. Accessed September 28, 2008, from the Association of Standardized Patient Educators website: http://www.aspeducators.org/sp_info.htm

Hofmeister, M. (April 20, 2007). *Medical admissions interviews.* Unpublished PHD candidacy paper.

Kales, H.C., DiNardo, A.R., Blow, F.C., McCarthy, J.F., Ignacio, R.V., & Riba, M.B. (2006). International medical graduates and the diagnosis and treatment of late-life depression. *Academic Medicine, 81(2)*, 171–75.

Kidd, M.R., & Zulman, A. (1994). Educational support for overseas-trained doctors. *Medical Journal of Australia, 160*, 73–75.

Ko, D.T., Austin, P.C., Chan, B.T.B., & Tu, J.V. (2005). Quality of care of international and Canadian medical graduates in acute myocardial infarction. *Archives of Internal Medicine, 165(4)*, 458–63.

Kvern, B. (2001). Teaching international medical graduates in family medicine residency programs. *Newsletter of the Section of Teachers of Family Medicine, 9(2)*, 7–9.

Lammers, S., & Verhey, A. (Eds.). (1998). *On moral medicine: Theological perspectives in medical ethics* (2nd ed.). Grand Rapids, MI: Wm. B. Eedermans Publishing.

Lupton, D. (1994). *Medicine as culture: Illness, disease and the body in Western societies.* London: Sage.

McGlynn, E.A., Asch, S.M., Adams, J., Keesey, J., Hicks, J., DeCristofaro, A., et al. (2003). The quality of health care delivered to adults in the United States. *New England Journal of Medicine, 348(26)*, 2635–45.

Medical Council of Canada. (n.d.). About the examinations. Accessed September 28, 2008, at http://www.mcc.ca/en/exams/

Oath of Hippocrates, Modified Geneva Version, World Medical Association. 1993.

Peitzman, S.J., McKinley, D., Curtis, M., Burdick, W., & Whelan, G. (2000). International medical graduates' performances of techniques of physical examination, with a comparison of U.S. citizens and non-U.S. citizens. *Academic Medicine, 75(10)*, s115–17.

Royal College of Physicians and Surgeons of Canada. (2009). International medical graduates. Accessed June 20, 2010, at http://rcpsc.medical.org/residency/certification/img_e.php

Sackett, D.L., Rosenberg, W.M.C., Gray, J.A.M., Haynes, R.B., & Richardson, W.S. (1996). Evidence based medicine: What it is and what it isn't. *British Medical Journal, 312(7023)*, 71–72.

Sannoufi, H. (2004). *The challenges of international medical graduates in the Canadian health care system*. Unpublished manuscript, Dalhousie University, Halifax, NS, Canada.

Schuster, M.A., McGlynn, E.A., & Brook, R. (1998). How good is the quality of health care in the United States? *Milbank Quarterly, 76(4)*, 517–64.

Searight, H.R., & Gafford, J. (2006). Behavioural science education and the international medical graduate. *Academic Medicine, 81(2)*, 164–70.

Singhal, K., & Ramakrishnan, K. (2004). Training needs of international medical graduates seeking residency training: Evaluation of medical training in India and the United States. *Internet Journal of Family Practice, 3(1)*, http://www.ispub.com/ostia/index.php?xmlFilePath=journals/ijfp/vol3n1/img.xml

Steinert, Y., & Walsh, A. (Eds.). (2006). *Faculty development program for teachers of international medical graduates*. Accessed September 28, 2008, from the Association of Faculties of Medicine of Canada website: http://www.afmc.ca/img/default_en.htm

Sung, N.S., Crowley, W.F., Jr., Genel, M., Salber, P., Sandy, L., Sherwood, L.M., et al. (2003). Central challenges facing the national clinical research enterprise. *Journal of the American Medical Association, 289(10)*, 1278–87.

Szafran, O., Crutcher, R., Banner, S., & Watanabe, M. (2005). Canadian and immigrant international medical graduates. *Canadian Family Physician, 51(9)*, 1242–43, e1–e6.

World Health Organization. (2007, January). World directory of medical schools. Accessed September 28, 2008, at http://www.who.int/hrh/documents/wdms_upgrade/en/index.html

MAPPING DIVERSITY

THE CONTRIBUTION OF GEOGRAPHICAL INFORMATION SYSTEMS TO THE ALBERTA INTERNATIONAL MEDICAL GRADUATE PROGRAM

Chantal Hansen MGIS

Nigel Waters PhD

Luz Palacios-Derflingher PhD

Rodney A. Crutcher
MD, MMedEd, CCFP(EM)

INTRODUCTION

There are physician shortages provincially, nationally, and globally. There is a worldwide migration of physicians, generally from less-developed countries to those better developed. As one strategy to help address provincial workforce shortages, the Alberta International Medical Graduate (AIMG) Program was created to increase the number of IMGs practising medicine in the province. It does this by selecting and preparing Albertans who are graduates of World Health Organization–listed medical schools outside Canada or the United States for postgraduate medical residency training in high need specialties in Alberta.

Two of the AIMG Program's goals are communication and development. The communication goal includes keeping stakeholders informed of program processes, policies, and outcomes. The development goal has a quality improvement focus with a specific objective of supporting research, evaluation, and development activities that enhance the AIMG Program. Part of the AIMG Program's current research work is to increase the understanding of the socio-cultural characteristics of IMGs applying to, and accepted by, the program.

It is clear that AIMG Program applicants are heterogeneous. A review of the AIMG database reveals that applicants' demographic and educational data varies in many areas: the country and system of medical education; the duration and content of training; clinical experience during and after training; and interpersonal competencies as assessed during the AIMG Program's admissions interview procedures.

Of central interest to the AIMG Program is the answer to the question: "What are the characteristics of a successful AIMG Program applicant?" This knowledge is important to AIMG Program policy and practice and may also contribute to health workforce theory.

The AIMG Program's desire to explore state-of-the-art approaches to data display and hypothesis generation has led it to the use of Geographic Information Systems (GIS) technology. GIS methodologies such as mapping and analysis are valuable tools in understanding the nature of, the relationships with, and the interactions between many variables. In the AIMG Program, GIS techniques have been used to geo-code data, display selected applicant characteristics, and explore country-specific correlations between country of medical degree, applicant success, and the general population immigrating to Alberta.

THE GIS ADVANTAGE

Geographic Information Systems are computer-based decision support systems that link geographic information with descriptive information (Longley, Goodchild, Maguire, & Rhind, 2005). GIS provide a technology and methodology to explore and analyze spatial data, or information about the earth, its people, and the spaces within which they move. Recognizing this "context" (setting or environment) means people can be linked to place— and this means that the "where" that is critical to an event, behaviour, or phenomenon may be identified. Often the "why" depends on the "where." With the advent of sophisticated technology and new methodologies of spatial analysis (such as GIS, global positioning systems, remote sensing, and spatial statistics), researchers are paying increased attention to location and spatial interaction in their theoretical frameworks (Goodchild, Anselin, Appelbaum, & Harthorn, 2000). GIS analysis has several advantages over traditional approaches: (1) it allows the integration of independent data sets; (2) it provides visual and spatial presentation of the data and relationships that exist; and (3) it allows exploratory and confirmatory spatial analysis.

Increasingly, data on human populations and their socio-demographic characteristics are being integrated into GIS databases.[1] This "geo-demographic" analysis of populations by place of residence, exploring composition, events, activities, and how they are distributed, demonstrates the relevance of GIS for the AIMG Program. Using GIS, the AIMG Program can determine how a particular phenomenon (in this case program applicant success) relates to selected demographic and educational variables such as ethnicity, gender, duration of medical school training, examination results, and country of medical education.

To date, in the AIMG Program, GIS has been primarily used as a visualization tool. It readily provides a holistic picture of AIMG applicants. GIS enables the program to see where the applicants were trained, what is happening over time with each new cohort, and the importance of other social and cultural variables that, until now, have only been comprehended anecdotally. This is significant because, in turn, this analysis may provide important insights about IMG education, and may thus influence AIMG policy, practice, and research activities. GIS complements more traditional data tools, including commonly available statistical software packages: the spatial images are powerful and can be readily assimilated by expert and non-expert alike. This is not true for traditional multivariate analyses, which produce complex, difficult-to-interpret statistical artifacts. While the GIS analyses are indeed just another way of looking at the applicant data, the different view provided by GIS may likely yield dramatically different insights into the structure of the data. From the AIMG Program perspective, using GIS compared to traditional data tools is not a matter of "if/or" but rather "both/and."

GIS FOR SOCIO-CULTURAL EXPLORATIONS: A LITERATURE REVIEW

The increased use of GIS as an assessment and evaluation tool and as a visual aid has enabled researchers to begin to explore human populations and their various social characteristics through spatial analysis. Although GIS technologies are now being utilized to analyze social processes and characteristics, most of the literature to date focuses on GIS applications for the mapping and analysis of population characteristics for marketing, crime, and public health.[2]

GIS may be used to explore socio-cultural patterns among different groups of people. While there have been major advances in the use of GIS for socio-cultural studies of populations, there are relatively few published discussions of these new applications and their use in broadening our understanding of why phenomena are occurring. Aldenderfer and Maschner (1996) explore GIS applications in cultural anthropology, archaeology, paleoanthropology, and physical anthropology, and their book is one of only a small number to focus on GIS for cultural investigations. To date, papers that explore GIS and socio-cultural characteristics of populations have focused on archaeological analysis (Brandt, Groenewoudt, & Kvamme, 1992; Robbins, 1984), Indigenous communities and their interaction with the land (Clayton & Waters, 1999; Chapin, Lamb, & Threlkeld, 2005), linguistic differences among communities (Dow, 1994) and, recently, military applications known as human terrain systems (Schaefer, 2006; González, 2008). Thus, the innovative application of GIS for exploring the socio-cultural contexts within the IMG population is apparent.

To date, much has been written about the cultural differences of IMGs (Fiscella, Roman-Diaz, Lue, Botelho, & Frankel, 1997; Kvern, 2001; Majumdar, Keystone, & Cuttress, 1999), and the needs of IMGs (Kvern, 2001; Hall, Keely, Dojeiji, Byszewski, & Marks, 2004; Kidd & Zulman 1994). Pilotto, Duncan, and Anderson-Wurf (2007) provide a systematic review of papers listed on the MEDLINE database for the period 1990–2006 that address cultural issues encountered in IMG programs. These articles discuss in detail IMG gender, age, education, and ethnicity—and use traditional (aspatial) statistics to calculate and compare differences among IMG groups. These aspatial techniques present only part of the story. Almost all human activities and decisions involve an important geographic component—they are located on the earth's surface and this location is in itself analytically useful. It is essential to incorporate this variable and thus utilize spatial analysis techniques *as well* in the data analyses. Location can integrate socio-cultural information about IMGs and facilitate the interpretation of complex interdependent relationships. At specific places and times, demographic, cultural, and other social processes combine and interact, and the implementation of GIS and spatial analysis can provide the key to a greater understanding of these interactions (Goodchild et al., 2000). Audas, Ross, and Vardy (2004) state that country of origin (and medical education), among other characteristics of IMGs entering Canada, is a grossly understudied area of human health resources. This variable forms the context for the GIS mapping of the AIMG Program applicants.

Relevant to investigations linked to country of medical education is the association with immigration. Canada has been the beneficiary of large-scale immigration of physicians over the past half century (Mejia & Pizurki, 1976; Mullan, Politzer, & Davis, 1995). Medical training positions in Alberta, as well as opportunities for medical employment, have proved a strong draw for physicians from many nations. Despite the large number of unlicensed international medical graduates living in Canada, comparative data on the numbers or national origins of these physicians have not been available.

GIS AND THE AIMG PROGRAM

The creation and application of GIS provides a rich research tool for visualizing and exploring spatial relationships in the AIMG applicant database. The AIMG dataset contains location-based information: country of birth, country of medical education, and city of current residence. Mapping the AIMG database provides context and conveys perspective. Displaying visual representations of the AIMG data assists researchers and policy-makers in generating ideas and hypotheses about the data. Vital spatial patterns are easily concealed in documents, charts, or spreadsheets, but with the common reference of location, it is easy and effective to represent, integrate, and access information through geography. Importantly, data from other sources such as the World Health Organization's Directory of Medical Schools and Statistics Canada immigration statistics may be integrated with the GIS to gain further insight from the collected AIMG Program data.

The following maps are the result of combining the AIMG Program database (402 application records from individuals in 53 countries) for the period 2001 to 2006 with Environmental Systems Research Institute's spatial dataset containing the countries of the world. Presenting data in the form of a map helps users understand the significance of where IMGs are applying from, identify the characteristics of IMGs from different countries, and visualize patterns or relationships inherent in the IMG applicant pool.

Total AIMG Applicants, 2001–2006

The GIS was used to generate choropleth maps that displayed the percentage of AIMG applicants for the period 2001–2006. Choropleth maps

FIGURE 1: *Country of Medical School Education for All Applicants*
(colour image p. 293)

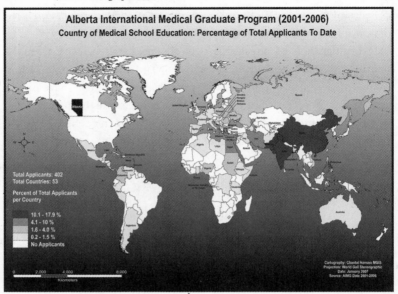

(Slocum, McMaster, Kessler, & Howard, 2005, pp. 250–70) are shaded in proportion to the value of the statistical variable displayed on the map; figure 1, for example, shows the percentage of AIMG applicants by their country of medical education. These maps provide an easy way to visualize how a measurement varies across a geographic area (country of medical education).

In figure 1, the darkness or lightness of a country is proportional to the percentage of all applicants for the years 2001–2006 who received their medical education there. Class division is based on natural breaks inherent in the data (McGrew & Monroe, 2000). Figure 1 shows that the predominant streams of program applicants originate from India, Pakistan, and China (43%), almost half of the total applicant pool; these nations are thus displayed with the darker shade indicating the higher concentration. Several countries (palest yellow) have less than five applicants and those that remain white had no applicants at all during this time period.

The power of a map is that it shows spatial patterns, if any such patterns exist. It is apparent that the countries with a high number of applicants are not random. Southern Asia and China have a much higher proportion of applicants than other countries of the world. Thus questions are raised: Why

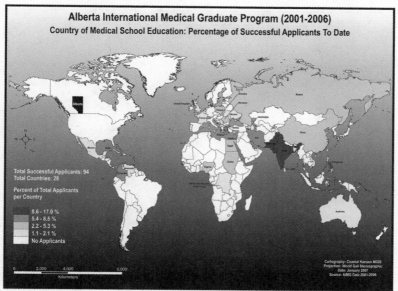

are so many IMGs with a medical education from these countries applying to the AIMG Program? Is there an underlying spatial process influencing this pattern? Is there a similar pattern among other IMG programs in other provinces? Is there a direct connection with immigration to Alberta and/or Canada?

Successful AIMG Applicants, 2001–2006

Figure 2 shows the countries from which the successful AIMG Program applicants obtained their medical education.

Pakistan and India provide the highest percentages of successful AIMG Program applicants (17% and 13% respectively). Although China also provides a significant number of program applicants, application success among these candidates is limited (4%). Displaying this information geographically is useful: while the majority of IMG applicants originate from these neighbouring and highly populated nations, arguably some of the oldest civilizations in Asia, applicants' chances of securing a position within the AIMG Program are quite different. This naturally invites further exploration of cultural differences (captured in the AIMG database) between these countries: language, education, and gender.

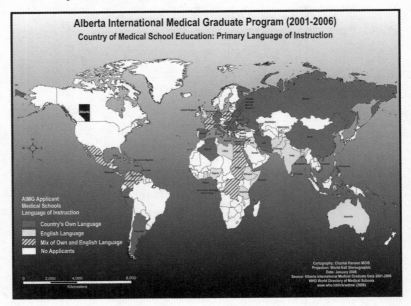

Language of Instruction

In explaining the distributions shown in figures 1 and 2, the success of applicants from Pakistan and India may reflect the fact that their medical schools are patterned after the British system of education, and testing and instruction occur in English (World Health Organization [WHO], 2006). Thus, the medical education system of these countries is somewhat similar to that of Canada. This requires further analysis to confirm, such as correlating data from other sources, analysis that is facilitated by the GIS. Figure 3 uses WHO data on international medical schools to display the primary language of instruction for AIMG Program applicant medical schools only, aggregated at the country level. No data is provided by WHO on which specific courses or subjects are taught in different languages, so this map is a generalization of the applicants' overall medical education.

It is readily apparent from cross-referencing the maps (figures 2 and 3) that countries with a high applicant success rate have English medical instruction (though some African countries with English medical instruction have not been successful, notably Ethiopia, Ghana, Libya, Somalia, and Tanzania—perhaps due to the small number of applicants from these countries). English language proficiency is clearly a factor in the AIMG Program selection process. All program applicants must demonstrate competence in written and spoken English. IMGs—no matter their country of medical degree—are often familiar with medical terms due to the common Latin roots, but English pronunciation and fluency can be difficult (Armson & Crutcher, 2006). Proficiency in the English language in a medical setting is a significant hurdle for some program applicants.

The system of medical education in China is very different from the system in North America, Western Europe, and former British colonies. As modern Western medical curricula have moved toward inquiry-based approaches to learning, emphasizing creativity, critical thinking, and the application of knowledge, the approach of Chinese medical educators remains for the most part influenced by a more authoritarian and didactic system of teaching, where expert opinion and the rote learning of facts prevail (Field, Geffen, & Walters, 2006). Both traditional Chinese medicine and traditional Mongolian medicine play a significant role in today's Chinese medical curriculum (Cooper & Yingang, 1987). Also, the nature of the patient–physician relationship varies substantially between Western and Chinese cultures. A relationship-oriented, patient-centred model, common in North America, is not the norm in China. Given the historical and colonial connections between India and Pakistan on the one hand, and Western Europe and Canada on the other, there are both greater cultural congruence and medical system "fit" in this area. The Chinese model of patient–physician relationships reflects Chinese Confucian cultural commitments, whereby a paternalistic attitude, which legitimizes the doctors' right to exert power over their patients, is the norm (Feldman, Zhang, & Cummings, 1999).

The ability to communicate goes beyond the capacity to speak and write English. Issues related to verbal and non-verbal communication skills, interpersonal skills, and other humanistic and cultural nuances are as important as medical knowledge and clinical skills. The extent to which the IMG can vary his or her own verbal and non-verbal responses and is able to say things in a way that a patient can understand and feel comfortable with does influence the IMG's likelihood of success in the program. Research suggests a link between the successful development

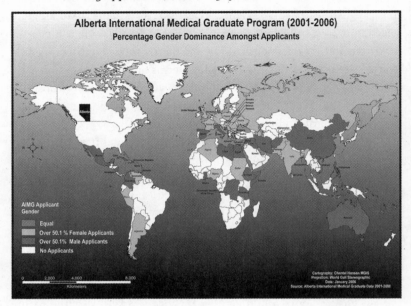

of patient–physician rapport and gender (Roter & Hall, 2004; Weisman & Teitelbaum, 1989). Thus, gender is another variable within the AIMG database that is mapped in the GIS.

Figure 4 shows the dominant gender of AIMG Program applicants. Countries with a dominant gender (equal to or greater than 50.1%) are displayed: male and female applicant dominance is shown using blue and orange respectively.

Immediately a pattern can be seen with our three focus countries: most IMGs that apply to the AIMG Program from China are male; most IMGs that apply from India and Pakistan are female. Linking this to the previous map of success in the AIMG Program (figure 2), exploring this limited applicant success for Chinese IMGs may invite questions: Why are there fewer female IMGs from China applying to the AIMG Program? Would the success rate for Chinese IMGs increase if more females applied to the AIMG Program?

Is this a culturally significant finding within the data? The Confucian ideology, which has been deeply rooted throughout Chinese history, confined females to an oppressed social status (Croll, 1977; Song, 2004). Acceptance of women in public educational settings, availability of educational opportunities for women, and equal treatment for female students are variables that affect women's entrance to schools in China (Liu & Carpenter, 2005)—including medical schools. While more than 50 years of socialist gender equality policies and practices have succeeded somewhat in promoting females' attendance in schools, an imbalance of educational opportunities and achievements for women still exists. As education in China becomes more equalized, the GIS maps may indeed present an entirely different picture once more female IMGs begin to apply.

Conversely, the opportunities for females to attend medical school in both India and Pakistan reflect the changing position of women in these countries. Recent social and political reforms have meant that women have had increased participation in public and professional life. An apt example is the profession of medicine itself—the treatment of Indian women by male physicians posed cultural problems, and female physicians filled a real need (Leonard, 1976). Thus, the higher percentage of female AIMG applicants graduating from medical schools in India and Pakistan is reflected in the GIS maps.

In relation to the gender of all applicants, the AIMG Program is uncertain as to the reasons for differential success rates during the admissions process. It has reviewed its processes and data, and has not found evidence of any systemic bias. There are consistent findings in the literature in that women tend to perform better than men in their medical training (Oggins, Inglehart, Brown, & Moore, 1988). Women also tend to perform better in clinical assessments (Weinberg & Rooney, 1973). The AIMG Program is aware that some IMGs resident in Alberta state that female IMGs trying to access a residency training position through the AIMG Program can stay home to study, where males may need to work outside of the home to support their family, and thus have limited time to study.

Trend over Time

By comparing data from two or more time periods, the GIS can be used to identify trends over time. By mapping where and how things fluctuate, the AIMG Program gains insight into how the applicant cohort changes. This is important to anticipate future needs, to decide on possible courses of action, and to evaluate the results of an action or policy. For example, if the AIMG dataset is compared between 2001 and 2006 (figures 5 and 6), the pattern generally remains consistent with the successful focus countries: India and Pakistan have a high percentage of applicants for both of those years.

FIGURE 5: *Country of Medical School Education for 2001 Applicants*
(colour image p. 295)

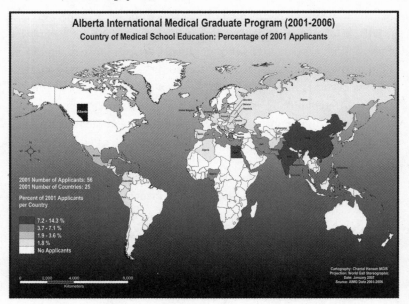

The percentage of applicants from China has dropped by 2006. Also, with the increasing number of applicants over time, there is a growing diversity among applicants' country of medical education.

This comparison poses important questions for policy-makers: How does the AIMG Program address the needs and expectations of IMGs trained in China? For Chinese Canadians, does having access to physicians who speak Chinese and have some cultural understanding of their health traditions and beliefs play an important role in the quality of their life? If this is the case, then the GIS maps have helped highlight the need for culturally competent care.

The AIMG Program recognizes that an increasingly diverse Albertan population poses challenges in the provision of culturally sensitive and culturally competent care[3] (Rogerson, 2006). In the U.S., physician leaders and educators believe that the diversity of the health professional workforce should mirror that of the population (Sullivan Commission, 2004). Canada does not have such explicit goals related to ethnicity, but the issue of ensuring that doctors can provide culturally competent care is high on the medical education agenda.

FIGURE 6: *Country of Medical School Education for 2006 Applicants*
(colour image p. 295)

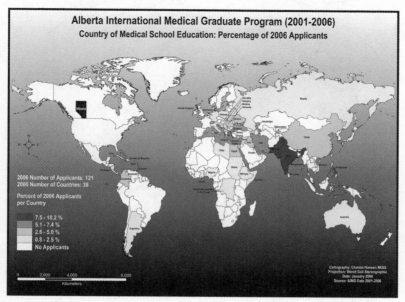

Given Albertan physician workforce shortages and the many unlicensed IMGs living in Alberta who wish to once more work at their chosen profession, it is important to examine the immigration patterns to Alberta to understand both the needs and the resource pool from which the AIMG Program has to draw. Qualified but currently unlicensed IMGs have the potential to contribute greatly to the health care needs of the Albertan public. As per AIMG Program policy, program applicants, no matter where they were educated, must be residents of Alberta or Canadian citizens to be eligible to apply.

Immigration Patterns to Alberta

To begin to understand the relationship between immigration patterns to Alberta and the characteristics of IMG program applicants, additional data incorporated into the GIS are Alberta's immigration statistics from Citizenship and Immigration Canada. In 1996, the top two source areas for immigrants to Alberta were the United Kingdom (15.2%) and other European countries (15.2%). Less than a decade later, in 2004, the top four source countries for immigration to Alberta were China (13.3%), the

FIGURE 7: *Immigration to Alberta 2004 (colour image p. 296)*

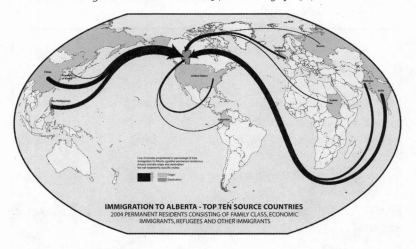

IMMIGRATION TO ALBERTA - TOP TEN SOURCE COUNTRIES
2004 PERMANENT RESIDENTS CONSISTING OF FAMILY CLASS, ECONOMIC
IMMIGRANTS, REFUGEES AND OTHER IMMIGRANTS

Philippines (12.0%), India (9.9%), and Pakistan (6.7%) (see figure 7). African immigrants have also increased in number since the mid-1990s. Not surprisingly, the countries from which AIMG applicants most frequently obtained their medical degrees reflect the sources of recent immigration to Alberta (Alberta Employment, Immigration, and Industry, 2005). This shift in the immigration pattern to Alberta has had unique impacts on the provision of culturally sensitive care required in the province. Indeed, IMGs from the current primary source countries seeking a licence to practise would provide more "accessible" health care to Canadian patients with the same ethno-cultural background.

Burgeoning research has indicated that there is a certain degree of "spatial mismatch" between immigrant health care demand and the supply of culturally diverse physicians. A recent study out of Toronto points to the need for Canada's health care system to recognize the cultural and language barriers that immigrants face when seeking primary care physicians who understand the beliefs and values unique to their ethnicity. Canada (including Alberta) needs to better address issues relating to training and licensing of foreign-trained physicians (Wang, 2007). A paucity of IMGs from China successfully accessing residency training through the AIMG Program (figure 2) suggests the possibility of spatial inequality among Chinese immigrants in accessing culturally sensitive health care.

QUANTITATIVE ANALYSES

The maps presented above have raised some interesting questions regarding differences between IMGs from China and India, and thus have enabled the AIMG Program to take a more focused approach with traditional statistical testing. One of the hypotheses of interest is to understand which charac-teristics may be of relevance to a successful application. As the GIS maps in figures 1 and 2 reveal, country of medical school education is emphasized as a characteristic of importance in successful applications (i.e., completing a medical degree in India tends to lead to more success than completing one in China).

The applicants to the AIMG Program go through several stages during the application process. They need to satisfy several requirements, such as completion of a medical degree from a WHO-recognized medical school (outside Canada and the U.S.) and proof of residence in Alberta. Later, they are invited to an Objective Structured Clinical Examination (OSCE), and once they have ranked well in this stage, they are invited for an interview.[4] The following analyses were performed with data from the IMG applicants who applied to family medicine and who satisfied these requirements (i.e., they were granted an interview).

Univariate Analyses

Univariate analyses comparing medical school country with one character-istic at a time (in this case China and India) were performed for the years 2002 to 2006 (44 applications: 15 from China and 29 from India).[5] While univariate analysis can be used to better understand how each character-istic differs or is equal with respect to the two countries, it will not provide a complete picture since other characteristics may also be of influence in the outcome. Chi-squared tests and t-tests were performed where deemed appropriate (Field, 2005). Table 1 shows the number of applications accepted by country for the period 2002–2006. After performing a test of independ-ence, it can be concluded that the proportion of applications accepted is not significantly different for the two countries.

In China, the proportion of success is 20% with a 95% confidence inter-val (CI)[6] (4.33%, 48.08%), and in India the proportion of success is 44.82% with a 95% CI (26.44%, 64.30%).[7]

As can be seen in table 2, the proportion of applicants who were male or female is not the same in the different countries. Again, a test of

TABLE 1: *AIMG Program Acceptance by Country (2002–2006) for Applicants After the Interview Process*

Accepted	China	India	Total
No	12	16	28
Yes	3	13	16
Total	15	29	44

independence was performed. The proportion of males in China is 73.30% with a 95% CI (44.89%, 92.21%), and the proportion of males in India is 20.68% with 95% CI (7.99%, 39.72%).

TABLE 2: *Gender by Country (2002–2006) for AIMG Program Applicants After the Interview Process*

Gender	China	India	Total
Female	4	23	27
Male	11	6	17
Total	15	29	44

Table 3 shows a clear, lopsided difference in language of instruction between the two countries.

TABLE 3: *Language of Instruction by Country (2002–2006) for AIMG Program Applicants After the Interview Process*

Language of instruction:	China	India	Total
No English	12	0	12
Only English	0	22	22
English and others	3	5	8
Total	15	27	42

Note: The total number of applications here differs from the previous total (44), because two applications had missing values.

After performing tests of equality of the means for OSCE scores, year of graduation, and interview scores between China and India, it can be concluded that OSCE scores are not different, and that year of graduation and interview scores are different between the two countries. Box plots[8] (Field, 2005) of these three characteristics, by country, can be seen in figures 8, 9, and 10.

FIGURE 8: *OSCE Scores by Country (2002–2006) for AIMG Program Applicants Who Went on to the Interview Process*

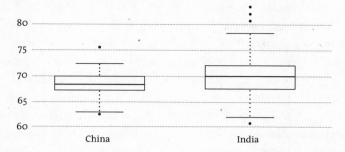

FIGURE 9: *Year of Graduation by Country (2002–2006) for AIMG Program Applicants Who Went on to the Interview Process*

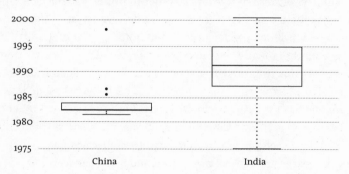

FIGURE 10: *Interview Scores by Country (2002–2006) for AIMG Program Applicants Who Went on to the Interview Process*

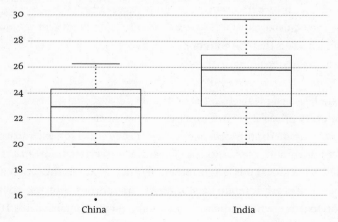

Univariate tests do not provide a complete understanding as other variables may influence the outcome. In order to obtain a model that can incorporate more than one characteristic at the same time and that could indicate which characteristics are of importance, a regression analysis may be employed. Since the outcome variable is dichotomous (success / no success), a logistic regression analysis was performed (Hosmer, 2000). In this type of regression, one can calculate the probability and odds ratio (ratio of odds) of acceptance.

Logistic Regression

The data analyzed comprises the period 2002 to 2006 (165 applications) for all the countries. The sample size was not large enough to be able to perform an analysis that would take into account influences from each different country. Because of this and in order to preserve some geographical representation, countries were grouped into seven zones.[9] The characteristics studied included gender, duration in training, year of graduation, English as a mother tongue, overall OSCE score, language of instruction, medical school country (grouped), and interview score. To illustrate, a simple analysis that incorporated only the effect of each characteristic in an additive manner on the response (main effect) in the presence of other characteristics was performed. No interacting characteristics (interactions) were included in the analysis. The characteristics discovered to be of importance were year of graduation, OSCE score, and interview score.

The adjusted odds ratio[10] for year of graduation is 1.1036 (95% CI [1.0400, 1.1711]), which means that the odds of being accepted increase 1.1036 times for every increase of one year in graduation year. Simply stated, more recent graduates have better odds of program acceptance.

The adjusted odds ratio for OSCE score is 1.1143 (95% CI [1.0239, 1.2126]), which means that the odds of being accepted increase 1.1143 times for every increase of one point in OSCE score.

The adjusted odds ratio for interview score is 1.8576 (95% CI [1.4892, 2.3171]), which means that the odds of being accepted increase 1.8576 times for every increase of one point in interview score.

The predicted probability of acceptance for a person with an OSCE score of 69.4, a year of graduation of 1991, and an interview score of 24.75 (median values of the data) is 0.4517 (95% CI [0.3544, 0.5529]). Thus, the traditional statistical analyses employed to draw inferences about the IMG population together with the patterns highlighted by the maps enabled the AIMG

Program to predict the profile of IMGs with certain cultural and socio-demographic characteristics being accepted into the program.

LIMITATIONS

The GIS work for the AIMG Program does have some limitations. Mapping at the country level means that the data are aggregated to their fullest extent and the ecological fallacy comes into effect. The ecological fallacy is the inappropriate inference of individual relationships from areal unit results (Wrigley, Holt, Steel, & Tranmer, 1996). Any observed pattern in the mapped data may be due to the particular configuration of zonal boundaries used; the relationship between variables that are observed at one level of aggregation may not hold at the individual or any other level of aggregation (Martin, 1996). Much research has been conducted about this issue including Openshaw's research (1984), in which he quantified the typical range of ecological fallacy problems that might be expected in census data analysis. In this case, we are simply providing a holistic view of the IMGs to see general patterns by country.

All applications are considered unique, even if subjects applied more than once for each year. This could introduce a bias in both the GIS and logistic regression analysis, especially for those characteristics that do not change (i.e., medical school country and gender). The words "applicants" and "applications" are used interchangeably.

CONCLUSION

The Alberta International Medical Graduate (AIMG) Program has initiated the use of GIS to map the socio-cultural characteristics of their IMG applicant pool. The maps and research facilitated by GIS have helped to suggest possible causes of the observed geographic patterns. There are culturally significant variables within the AIMG database that invite further analysis. Knowing the IMG's country of medical education and how different cultures affect IMG gender, education, language, and examination results helps to explain the success rates of applicants from different countries.

Mapping different phenomena and having the ability to integrate disparate data enables researchers to cut through noise and complexity to get straight to potentially meaningful trends and patterns. GIS has long been recognized as a technology that can help cross borders and see the whole by integrating information into a common spatial and visual language. Importantly for the AIMG Program, this generates discussion—the appeal of an intriguing and innovative display cannot be underestimated. Quantitative analyses add traditional statistical rigour to the observed patterns presented by the maps. Predictors of admission success for the 2001–2006 AIMG applicant cohort provide important information for program processes, policies, and outcomes.

These multi-method approaches (thematic maps, flow maps, statistics, and spatial analyses) have been helpful to the AIMG Program's goals. We hope they are also of interest to others in the health workforce, medical education, and broader academic communities.

Disclaimer: The views above are those of the authors and do not necessarily reflect the view of Alberta Health and Wellness or the Alberta International Medical Graduate Program.

NOTES

1. See Longley et al. (2001), Okabe (2005), and Harris, Sleight, and Webber (2005) for examples of GIS applications on census and customer data.
2. These vast subjects are beyond the scope of this chapter; please refer to Harris et al. (2005), Chainey and Ratcliffe (2005), and Cromley and McLafferty (2002), among others.
3. In Calgary alone, it has been recently estimated that there are over 90 distinct ethnic groups (Statistics Canada, 2007).
4. The interview portion of the selection process (conducted in English) is designed for the AIMG Program to learn more about the candidate's qualities as they relate to being a good physician and the suitability of the candidate for postgraduate training.
5. 2001 applicants were not included due to the significant change in structure of the interview process.
6. A 95% confidence interval (CI) gives plausible values for the population's proportion. Given that some of the procedures used in the process for constructing such intervals are prone to the effects of chance, the interval correctly contains, in general, the true value of the proportion 95% of the time.
7. The CIs overlap appreciably, and it is unlikely that the two percentages are significantly different.
8. The box plot is a graphical representation of data for showing simultaneous comparisons. These plots consist of three components: 1) the box, which encompasses the middle 50% of the data; 2) the horizontal line within the box, which represents the median value; and 3) the vertical lines extending above and below the box, which are 1.5 times the interquartile range (the interquartile range is the difference between the third quartile and the first quartile). The dots beyond the lines are the outliers.

9. Zoning was based on the United Nations Statistics Division's macro geo-graphical (continental) regions and geographical subregions: Africa, Latin America and the Caribbean, North America, Eastern and Western Europe, Asia, Oceania (2007).

10. The odds ratio compares the likelihood (as defined by odds) of a certain event between two groups. When expressing adjusted odds ratios, interpretation is based on comparing two subjects that have all other characteristics the same, regardless of the actual value, except for the characteristic of interest.

REFERENCES

Alberta. (2005, July 15). *Supporting immigrants and immigration to Alberta.* Edmonton: Human Resources and Employment. Accessed June 30, 2007, from Alberta Employment and Immigration website: http://employment.alberta.ca/documents/WIA/WIA-IM_policy_framework.pdf

Aldenderfer, M., & Maschner, H.D.G. (1996). *Anthropology, space and geographic information systems.* New York: Oxford University Press.

Armson, H., & Crutcher, R. (2006, April). *Orienting teachers and international medical Graduates: Part A: Orienting teachers: Understanding the IMGs' world; Part B: Orienting IMGs: Understanding the Canadian health care system and learning environment.* Ottawa: Association of Faculties of Medicine of Canada. Accessed November 16, 2007, from Association of Faculties of Medicine of Canada website: http://www.afmc.ca/img/pdf/OTI_en.pdf

Audas, R., Ross, A., & Vardy, D. (2004). *International medical graduates in Atlantic Canada.* Halifax, NS: Metropolis Atlantic.

Brandt, R., Groenewoudt, B.J., & Kvamme, K.L. (1992). An experiment in archaeo-logical site location: Modeling in the Netherlands using GIS techniques. *World Archaeology, 24,* 268–82.

Chainey, S., & Ratcliffe, J. (2005). *GIS and crime mapping.* London: John Wiley.

Chapin, M., Lamb, Z., & Threlkeld, B. (2005). Mapping indigenous lands. *Annual Review of Anthropology, 34,* 619–38.

Clayton, D., & Waters, N. (1999). Distributed knowledge, distributed processing, distributed users: Integrating case-based reasoning and GIS for multicriteria decision making. In J. Thill (Ed.), *Multicriteria decision-making and analysis: A geographic information sciences approach* (pp. 275–308). Brookfield: Ashgate.

Cooper, J.A., & Yingang, L. (1987). Medical education in People's Republic of China. *Journal of Medical Education, 62(4),* 287–304.

Croll, E. (1977). A recent movement to redefine the role and status of women. *China Quarterly, 71,* 591–97.

Dow, J.W. (1994). Anthropology: The mapping of cultural traits from field data. *Social Science Computer Review, 12(4),* 479–92.

Environmental Systems Research Institute. 2010. Accessed June 20, 2010, at http://www.esri.com

Feldman, M., Zhang, J., & Cummings, S. (1999). Chinese and U.S. internists adhere to different ethical standards. *Journal of General Internal Medicine, 14(8),* 469–73.

Field, A. (2005). Discovering statistics using SPSS (2nd ed.). London: Sage.

Field, M., Geffen, L., & Walters, T. (2006). Current perspectives on medical education in China. *Medical Education, 40(10)*, 938–39.

Fiscella, K., Roman-Diaz, M., Lue, B.H., Botelho, R., & Frankel, R. (1997). "Being a foreigner, I may be punished if I make a small mistake": Assessing transcultural experiences in caring for patients. *Family Practice, 14(2)*, 112–16.

González, R.J. (2008). Human terrain: Past, present and future applications. *Anthropology Today 24(1)*, 21–26.

Goodchild, M.F., Anselin, L., Appelbaum, R.P., & Harthorn, B.H. (2000). Toward spatially integrated social science. *International Regional Science Review, 23(2)*, 139–59.

Hall, P., Keely, E., Dojeiji, S., Byszewski, A., & Marks, M. (2004). Communication skills, cultural challenges and individual support: Challenges of international medical graduates in a Canadian healthcare environment. *Medical Teacher, 26(2)*, 120–25.

Harris, R., Sleight, P., & Webber, R. (2005). *Geodemographics, GIS and neighbourhood targeting*. Etobicoke, ON: John Wiley & Sons.

Hosmer, D.W., & Lemeshow, S. (2000). *Applied Logistic Regression* (2nd ed.). New York: Wiley-Interscience.

Kidd, M.R., & Zulman, A. (1994). Educational support for overseas-trained doctors. *Medical Journal of Australia, 160(2)*, 73–75.

Kvern, B. (2001). Teaching international medical graduates in family medicine residency programs. *Newsletter of the Section of Teachers of Family Medicine, 9(2)*, 7–9.

Leonard, K. (1976). Women and social change in modern India. *Feminist Studies, 3(3–4)*, 117–30.

Liu, J., & Carpenter, M. (2005). Trends and issues of women's education in China. *Clearing House: A Journal of Educational Strategies, Issues and Ideas, 78(6)*, 277.

Longley, P.A., Goodchild, M.F., Maguire, D.J., & Rhind, D.W. (2001). *Geographic information systems and science*. Hoboken, NJ: John Wiley & Sons.

———. (2005). *Geographic information systems and science* (2nd ed.). Chichester, U.K.: John Wiley & Sons.

Majumdar, B., Keystone, J.S., & Cuttress, L.A. (1999). Cultural sensitivity training among foreign medical graduates. *Medical Education, 33(3)*, 177–84.

Martin, D. (1996). An assessment of surface and zonal models of population. *International Journal of Geographical Information Systems*, 10, 973–89.

Mejia, A., & Pizurki, H. (1976). World migration of health manpower. *WHO Chronicle, 30(11)*, 455–60.

Mullan, F., Politzer, R.M., & Davis, C.H. (1995). Medical migration and the physician workforce: International medical graduates and American medicine. *Journal of the American Medical Association, 273(19)*, 1521–27.

McGrew, J.C., & Monroe, C.B. (2000). *An introduction to statistical problem solving in geography*. Boston: McGraw-Hill.

Oggins, J., Inglehart, M., Brown, D., & Moore, W. (1988). Gender differences in the prediction of medical students' clinical performance. *Journal of the American Medical Women's Association, 43*, 171–75.

Okabe, A. (2005). *Studies in human and social sciences with GIS*. Boca Raton, FL: CRC.

Openshaw, S. (1984). *The modifiable areal unit problem: Concepts and techniques in modern geography* (No. 38). Norwich: Geo Books.

Pilotto, L.S., Duncan, G.F., & Anderson-Wurf, J. (2007). Issues for clinicians training international medical graduates: A systematic review. *Medical Journal of Australia, 187(4)*, 225–28, http://www.mja.com.au/public/issues/187_04_200807/pil10257_fm.pdf

Robbins, C. (1984). Computer-assisted mapping. *Practicing Anthropology, 6(2)*, 15.

Rogerson, M. (2006). Cultural competence for practitioners: Diversity in practice; Becoming culturally competent. *WellSpring, 17(4)*. Accessed June 30, 2007, from the Alberta Centre for Active Living website: http://www.centre4activeliving.ca/publications/wellspring/2006/oct-culture.pdf

Roter, D.L., & Hall, J.A. (2004). Physician gender and patient-centered communication: A critical review of empirical research. *Annual Review of Public Health, 25*, 497–519.

Schaefer, P.W. (2006, August). *Mapping the human terrain: GIS in support of cultural intelligence*. Paper presented at the ESRI Users Conference held in San Diego, CA. Accessed June 20, 2010, from the Environmental Systems Research Institute website: http://proceedings.esri.com/library/userconf/proc06/papers/abstracts/a1048.html

Slocum, T.A., McMaster, R.B., Kessler, F.C., & Howard, H.H. (2005). *Thematic cartography and geographic visualization* (2nd ed.). Upper Saddle River, NJ: Pearson Education.

Song, G. (2004). *The fragile scholar: Power and masculinity in Chinese culture*. Hong Kong: Hong Kong University Press.

Statistics Canada. (2007). Selected ethnic origins, for census subdivisions (municipalities) with 5,000-plus population—20% sample data. Accessed June 30, 2007, at http://www12.statcan.ca/english/census01/products/highlight/ETO/Table1.cfm?T=501&Lang=E&GV=4&GID=4806016&Prov=48&S=0&O=A

Sullivan Commission. (2004). *Missing persons: Minorities in the health professions; A report of the Sullivan Commission on Diversity in the Healthcare Workforce*. Durham, NC: Sullivan Commission. Accessed June 30, 2007, at http://www.jointcenter.org/healthpolicy/docs/SullivanExecutiveSummary.pdf

United Nations Statistics Division. (2007). Composition of macro geographical (continental) regions, geographical sub-regions, and selected economic and other groupings. Accessed August 18, 2007, at http://unstats.un.org/unsd/methods/m49/m49regin.htm

Wang, L. (2007). Immigration, ethnicity, and accessibility to culturally diverse family physicians. *Health & Place, 13*, 656–71.

Weinberg, E., & Rooney, J. (1973). The academic performance of women students in medical school. *Journal of Medical Education, 48*, 240–47.

Weisman, C.S., & Teitelbaum, M.A. (1989). Women and health care communication. *Patient Education and Counselling, 13*, 183–99.

World Health Organization [WHO]. (2006). World directory of medical schools. Accessed September 28, 2008, at http://www.who.int/hrh/documents/wdms_upgrade/en/index.html

Wrigley, N., Holt, T., Steel, D., & Tranmer, M. (1996). Analysing, modelling, and resolving the ecological fallacy. In P. Longley & M. Batty (Eds.), *Spatial analysis: Modeling in a GIS environment* (pp. 25–40). Cambridge: GeoInformation International.

STORIES OF SEVEN
THE JOURNEY

INTERNATIONAL MEDICAL
GRADUATES IN CANADA

Gayle E. Rutherford RN, MN, PhD

INTERNATIONAL MEDICAL GRADUATES (IMGs) preparing to enter medical practice in Canada are faced with multiple challenges as they work toward reaching their goal. There are many IMGs in Alberta and Canada who want to practise medicine in their new country. We understand little about the IMG experience. This study was undertaken to begin to fill this gap.

The story of the journey of IMGs in Canada comes from stories gathered during telephone interviews with 16 IMGs preparing to enter medical practice in Alberta. These 16 IMGs responded to an electronic request for interviews sent in November 2003 to the 34 applicants for the 2002 Alberta International Medical Graduate (AIMG) Program. This study received ethics approval from the University of Calgary Conjoint Research Ethics Board. The researcher and participants reviewed a written informed consent form at the beginning of the telephone conversation and the participants' verbal consent to participate was recorded at the beginning of the interview conversations. The questions guiding the semi-structured conversational interviews focused on the background of the IMG, the experience of working toward becoming a practising physician in Canada, what has helped, and what has made it difficult. The interviews were conducted during November and December 2003. All interviews were conducted in English. For the most part, language was not a barrier during the interviews. The interviews were audiotaped and transcribed verbatim. The researcher performed initial data clustering and theme development using a NUD*IST qualitative data analysis software program.

The researcher was struck by the willingness of the IMGs to share their stories and by their determination to reach their goal of becoming a practising physician in Canada. Ten of the interviewees were female and six were male. Six were currently in family medicine residency programs. Their countries of origin were Pakistan (5), India (2), China (2), Poland (2), Columbia (2), Romania (1), Sudan (1), and Nigeria (1). The number of years each interviewee had been in Canada ranged from 4 to 11 with an average of 6.2 years. All interviewees obtained their basic medical training in their home country. Thirteen IMGs reported their years of practice as a general practitioner or family physician in their home countries as ranging from 0 to 9 years with an average of 3 years. Three IMGs had practiced within specialties for 1 to 10 years with an average of 4.3 years. Fourteen IMGs entered Canada as landed immigrants and two arrived as refugees. Twelve interviewees entered Canada with their families. All content in this story is based on interview data.

THE PUSH AND PULL OF A DREAM

Becoming a practising physician in Canada was very important to all of the IMGs. They spoke about their dream to be a doctor and how hard they were working to reach that dream. They talked about medicine as being their whole life until they came to Canada, and one stated that "it is very hard to give up, it is almost addictive." Practising medicine was like something coming from inside of them—a "fire within." They spoke about their passion for medicine and how from their earliest memory they had wanted to be doctors. They knew they had the skills to be physicians, they wanted to have those skills recognized, and they wanted to be able to use those skills to be with patients and to help them solve their problems. Practising medicine was part of who they were, and they found it very hard to give that up.

Before entering Canada, some of the IMGs had been aware of the challenges they would face when trying to practise medicine and others had

not. IMGs' stories included being told that they would not be able to practise medicine in Canada, but they had to make the choice to immigrate for
the welfare of their family: "the welfare of my family was, I put it above my
profession." They talked being told not to put their profession as a doctor or
"you wouldn't be allowed to immigrate so I came in as a homemaker." One
had to sign a paper to confirm that she would not practise medicine until
she had met the Canadian requirements and that she could not take any
action against the government if she did not get a job in the medical profession. Others were aware that it would be difficult to practise medicine in
Canada. They knew that they would have to write exams but had not been
aware of the challenges they would face after they had passed the exams.
Still others were surprised by the difficulties they faced. One IMG said he
met some physicians after he arrived in Canada who told him "this is very
tough, it's almost impossible, you better off even go to States." He did not
want to believe that.

After arriving in Canada, life changed significantly for some of the
IMGs, and their comments indicate the dichotomy between the positive
and the negative aspects of these changes. Adapting to a new culture was
difficult and exciting all at the same time. Arriving in a new country and
not knowing anyone outside of the immediate family could be very lonely:
"I was very lonely and alone in the world, as a doctor." Being exposed to the
Western world meant learning everything from the beginning. In some
ways it was exciting for women to learn they could be more independent in
Canada and do things they could not do at home. An IMG from Pakistan
said, "It is like being Alice in Wonderland or riding a bicycle for the first
time." They noted personal changes: "I'm more independent for myself....
more forward talking and not so shy." At the same time, the IMGs had to
step out and make an effort to meet people, to get to know the culture,
and to gain confidence in their use of the English language. Another interviewee from Pakistan spoke about not feeling that she has completed the
settlement process until she is able to practise medicine: "I still feel that I
am in the immigration process, from the bottom of my heart, although
I am a Canadian citizen of I think five years ago, six years ago, but still,
there is a part of me to be settled down."

THE EXAMS

IMGs must write and pass the Medical Council of Canada's Evaluating
Exam that tests basic medical knowledge before they are eligible to write

the medical qualifying exams written by Canadian medical graduates. When some of the IMGs wrote the Medical Council of Canada for information about the process of writing exam, they received an Evaluating Exam brochure that stated that there was very little chance for IMGs to get into a training program or to practise medicine in Canada. When asked if that was discouraging, one of the IMGs said, "Very, very, very, very." Some decided to study and write the exam even though they had no idea of what would happen after that. In 2000, these discouraging words were removed from the brochure. This was seen as a hopeful sign and a deciding factor for some IMGs to move forward with studying and writing exams. In order to apply for a residency position, the next step after passing the Evaluating Exam was to study for Part I of the Medical Council of Canada Qualifying Exam.

Making the decision to study for exams was not easy. IMGs had to find time to study while taking care of children and working "to help to make ends meet." This was particularly difficult without any extended family to turn to for support. The financial costs of writing exams were a barrier to some IMGs, particularly when there was always a risk of failure leading to duplication of these costs again in the future. IMGs had to pay a fee to write the exam and travel costs to get to the exam site. It was often not easy to get the money together or to get the time off from work. It was very difficult for IMGs who did not have a well-paying job or for those who had to work to support their families to raise the money to cover the costs and to find the time to study. There was no program for student financial assistance for IMGs to study for qualifying exams or to improve their English language skills. Those who had the financial support of a spouse were fortunate; they were able to use part of the income they got from their employment to cover the costs of the exams. Failure of an exam was "one of the lowest times" in the life of an IMG. When an IMG gets the results of the exam and "it is not what was expected, it is like a punch in the face." For some, the studying was different than they expected, and the exam was not what they imagined. For others, the English language caused some difficulty even though they felt they had the knowledge they needed to pass the exam. Those who passed the exam on the first try considered themselves to be truly fortunate.

In Canada, there is a system that matches medical graduates with placements for residency training across the country called the Canadian Resident Matching Service, or CaRMS for short. At the time of this study, IMGs were not eligible to apply to the first round of the match but could apply to the second round. For many, this was the only option they found to get into residency training. Residency training is required in order to get a licence to practise medicine in Canada. IMGs knew that they might be matched with any residency program across Canada, and this caused concern. Even with a supportive family, it would be hard to relocate everyone for the two years of residency training or to think about a family being separated for that length of time. It was a difficult decision to say that they would be willing to go anywhere because that was the only opportunity they had found to reach their dreams.

GETTING TO KNOW THE HEALTH CARE SYSTEM

IMGs spoke about how the actual practice of medicine is similar in Canada to their practice in their home countries. The basics of medicine do not change from country to country. Although the IMGs may have seen different illnesses in their home countries that are not common in Canada, they believed that there was not a big difference between what they learned in medical school and what they would be expected to do here. They recognized that there were more technological supports here to assist with the diagnostic and investigation processes and that they would need to learn more about these. At the same time, they believed that IMGs who have not had access to these advanced technologies have had to develop very strong clinical judgement skills to make diagnoses. The technology available here would actually make practising medicine easier. They looked forward to combining their clinical judgement skills with the technology available in Canada. Most importantly, they knew that they needed to learn more about the Canadian health care system and how the medical education system works in Canada.

Many IMGs in Alberta work in health-related fields and learn about the health care system through their work. These jobs varied from an office manager or receptionist in a medical clinic, to personal care or nursing aides, to research assistants or laboratory workers. Some are involved in full-time health-related careers such as acupuncture, chiropractic, or post-doctoral research. Working in health-related fields has provided many benefits to these IMGs. In many situations, they have had contact with patients and have had a chance to improve their English. It can be a challenge to understand what the patients want and to respond to their needs. Many of these jobs gave the IMGs an opportunity to meet practising physicians. Working within a medical clinic as a receptionist also helped an IMG to learn about the billing system, computers, and the paperwork involved in a family practice. The people IMGs worked with were often surprised to find out they were doctors, and some employers supported IMGs' need to take time to study or to observe physicians in practice.

CONNECTING WITH PHYSICIANS

The IMGs recognized the importance of connecting with physicians. Many IMGs had great difficulty making connection with physicians they could observe in practice and finding ways to get to know the health care system. It was very hard to make contacts when an IMG didn't know the system. Some IMGs were told to knock on doors and to keep knocking on doors until they found someone who would give them an opportunity to do an observership. Even though IMGs may have felt that their education was equal, they spoke about feeling "like an intruder" when they enter a practice environment requesting an opportunity to observe.

Some IMGs used the telephone directory to call doctor's offices and hospital departments, but found that physicians were already very busy with residents. Also, due to confidentiality or licensing issues, physicians were reluctant to have IMGs observe. Some IMGs were very persistent and eventually found an office or a department that would take them. IMGs call it the "lucky phone call." Others made connections through their own family physicians, and sometimes it took persistence to get the practising physician to really understand the barriers the IMG was facing. In general, practising physicians were quite supportive and the encouragement they provided was one of the most important factors that helped the IMGs to keep motivated to work toward their dream of once again practising medicine.

It was important to IMGs to have a formal observership set up with physicians where they could be directly involved with patients. They needed to practise taking patient histories and do physical examinations under the supervision of a practising physician. IMGs recognized that patients were different here because they were more educated and wanted to be more involved in the decisions about their treatment. Often, in their home countries, the patients just followed what the doctor said. Here, physicians needed to have really good communication skills and needed to continually be "on top of things, to do research and to find answers." Physicians have to be able to say things in a way that shows confidence and relays a message that the patient can be comfortable with. More hands-on practice increases an IMG's skills and improves his or her chances in applying to the AIMG Program.

THE AIMG PROGRAM APPLICATION PROCESS

The AIMG Program was formally established in 2001 to increase the number of IMGs who are eligible to work as medical doctors in Alberta. To IMGs in Alberta, this was the best news they had heard in a very long time. It was also a connection into a whole new world of opportunity. The IMGs were encouraged by the support of the people in the AIMG Program office and by the news that other IMGs had entered the program: "It was a booster" and "it motivated us to work harder" knowing that that could be them one day.

IMGs applying to the AIMG Program required reference letters from physicians. Those who had done observerships with physicians had little difficulty obtaining these reference letters. Those who had not made a connection with physicians in Alberta had to contact physicians in their home countries for reference letters. Each time an IMG applied to the AIMG Program, new reference letters were needed. This was very difficult for those who had no connection with physicians locally. If the IMG application was accepted, the IMG was invited to take an examination called the OSCE (Objective Structured Clinical Examination).

Many IMGs spoke about how the OSCE process was new to them and different from what they had experienced in their home countries. Comments on the OSCE indicated that this was a major hurdle for many. They talked about it being challenging because it was a clinical exam and it was so different to read about it than to do it. The IMGs found that they needed to behave like a student again rather than as someone who had practised as a physician. One IMG spoke about a surgical case where he knew very quickly what was going on and then forgot to ask all the questions and do all the tests that were required. The IMG later realized the need to ask questions and get the answers before making the diagnosis based on his past experiences. Language could cause difficulty for IMGs when taking the OSCE. They also need to use Canadian standards and practices in the OSCE rather than the standards of their own experiences. Working directly in observerships with physicians in practice and preparing together for the OSCE with other IMGs helped to increase the possibilities of passing this step in the AIMG Program. IMGs who passed the OSCE were invited to the next stage of an interview.

Some IMGs found the interview experience to be difficult. An IMG from Poland spoke about needing to learn "to sell myself and that is totally opposite to my culture" where "I had to be very modest, to show my papers, my diploma and shut my mouth." Whereas the IMG had learned that "If you talk too much, you know, you don't have much value in yourself," it was now important to overcome this habit and to learn how to "really push myself to tell about myself." As with the OSCE, each time IMGs went through the experience of an interview they gained skills and insights that would help them and others to be more successful on their next attempts. They also learned through these experiences that even though medicine may be similar everywhere, it is necessary to go through a training program in Canada to learn the specific ways of practising in Canada that are different from what they had been taught in their home countries.

The waiting period to find out if they had been accepted into the AIMG Program was long and stressful. The difficulty was that the number of IMGs applying to the AIMG Program was increasing every year, and it was getting harder to be accepted. IMGs spoke about their determination to keep on trying to get into a residency program, believing that "it was just a matter of time." As one IMG said, "I didn't tell those guys at the interview that I had with the AIMG but they will see me there until I get. They will see me at the AIMG Program until I will get in [sic]."

ALBERTA INTERNATIONAL MEDICAL GRADUATE ASSOCIATION

Some IMGs studied individually, but those who studied together with other IMGs found this provided them with much needed support. They felt they were not "alone anymore." It was helpful to study together and share knowledge, but it was also helpful to be with someone who was going through the same thing. They could learn from the experiences of those who had already passed exams and from those who had specialized knowledge in their fields of medicine. Joining a study group increased the possibility of passing exams on the first try. Even though the IMGs were competing for the same residency opportunities, they found that most shared freely of their knowledge and experiences for the mutual benefit of everyone in the group.

Some IMGs spoke about the importance of the Alberta International Medical Graduate Association (AIMGA) to them in their journey toward becoming a practising physician. In 2002, there were about 30 members. At the time of this study, there were over 100 member IMGs working toward becoming licensed to practise medicine in Alberta. The AIMGA brought together Albertan IMGs from all over the world with different experiences and backgrounds, enabling them to learn from each other. The IMG website received up to 15 emails each day. There was an increasing number of

IMGs who were beginning to take the exams and make connection through the AIMGA. Together they discussed exam questions, practised real patient scenarios in preparation for the OSCE, and prepared for interviews.

It is interesting to note that there were more female members than male members in the AIMGA—some said in a proportion of ten to one. Some IMGs speculated that this might be because more female doctors had entered Canada, often as the spouses of engineers or other professionals. It could also be that male physicians were the breadwinners in the family, and they were less likely to immigrate when there were few opportunities to enter medical practice. Male IMGs may also have less opportunity to take the time to study for exams because they need to work to feed their families. However, female IMGs sometimes felt like they had to work 24 hours a day to do everything that needed to get done. One IMG speculated that the imbalance between male and female IMGs in the AIMGA could be more related to the family situation than to whether the IMG is male or female. It could also relate to gender differences in seeking social support.

OBSERVERSHIP EXPERIENCE

Through the AIMGA, some of the IMGs had been able to get into an observership relationship. The Alberta Network of Immigrant Women was instrumental in making contact with doctors who were willing to accept IMGs. The IMGs rotated through these practices for three months at a time. The IMGs reported that the College of Physicians and Surgeons of Alberta was now willing to provide courtesy registration status for IMGs. This was an important step for IMGs because they could now take the history, do the physical examination and suggest a diagnosis when working with a preceptor, similar to the work that residents do in their training. A courtesy registration made a big difference in providing opportunities for IMGs to get hands-on Canadian experience, a definite advantage when applying for a residency position.

WHAT IMGS LEARNED

There is a need for more doctors in Alberta. If more IMGs have an opportunity to practise medicine, it will help to fill the need for more doctors and the IMGs will be able to provide important medical services for the increasingly diverse population in Alberta. The situation is improving and there seems to be more opportunity now than in the past, but it is very easy for an IMG to become discouraged. There is so much competition for so few positions. Some IMGs have applied through CaRMS and had interviews, but they were told that because there were so many candidates with such impressive backgrounds that they couldn't expect to get into a residency position. One person even thought about trying to go back into medical school but then thought, "How much farther behind am I going to start from?" IMGs are often underestimated and need to be given a chance. They are well-trained, intelligent, and diligent doctors who, with a little more training, can contribute to the health care system.

IMGs often wonder what makes a difference in the selection process. Some wonder if their age could be a factor. Are younger people chosen because they can practise for a longer time? Does an older IMG have an advantage due to maturity and experience? Will IMGs with a longer gap since practising medicine have difficulty updating their knowledge? They are clearly at a disadvantage compared to Canadian students who have continuity between medical school and residency training. Sometimes the gap in practice has been out of an IMG's control, especially if that IMG has been working toward entering practice the whole time. Language and ability to speak English well may also be a factor in the selection process. All applicants to the AIMG Program must pass an English language exam but they also need to be able to say things in a way that a patient can understand. IMGs are often familiar with medical terms due to the common Latin roots, but English pronunciation can be difficult.

Do some cultures have more advantages than others? IMGs have noted differences in acceptance based on their countries of origin. Some think that IMGs from English-speaking or European countries have advantages over those who are Asian. Chinese doctors in particular may have experienced greater challenges due to language and differences in the health care systems, because there is no system of family medicine within China. IMGs from some other countries are finding greater acceptance of their cultural differences. One IMG from Pakistan who wears a hijab said that this was not a barrier between her and her patients, and she was pleased that even though her patients were not from her culture, they understood. IMGs said that it is encouraging to see that doctors from a wider range of countries are getting in through the AIMG Program. Those who are in the program are opening doors for others from their home countries, and that is encouraging.

IMGs learned through listening to the IMGs who have already made it into a family medicine residency program. The AIMG Program's four-month orientation made a difference for those who enter through the program, and it was a good preparation for residency. IMGs in the AIMG Program reported that it is useful to have had some hospital experience as well as the family medicine practice experience before entering the program. It is important to learn about the role of medical clerks and residents in the hospital because this may be different from what an IMG has been used to and lack of familiarity with the Canadian medical education system makes it more difficult for IMGs. IMGs work very hard to fill their knowledge gaps during their training and sometimes need to work harder than the Canadian medical graduates. At other times, they have an advantage because of their past medical experiences. Confidence increases as the IMGs combine their new knowledge with their past skills. IMGs also reported that the benefits from the residency experience became clearer as time went on. An IMG from Nigeria said that once she started within the AIMG Program, she could see that there was no way she would have been prepared for the cultural differences in practice if she hadn't gone into a residency program.

ADVICE TO OTHER IMGS

This closing advice for IMGs evolved through interpretation of the IMG needs as told through their interview stories:

1. Build your personal support network. Studying and writing exams, gaining Canadian experience, and preparing to apply to the AIMG Program takes a lot of time and support. You will need cheerleaders who will give you encouragement to keep you going when you hit roadblocks along the way. If you have a family and children, you will need to have people who can help you with these responsibilities. Your spouse's support is essential.

2. Find opportunities to get to know the Canadian culture and to improve your English language skills. If you can, volunteering is a very good way to do this. If you have children in school, volunteer in your children's activities.

3. Talk about your dreams. Let people know that you are a doctor and that you want to become licensed to practise in Alberta. You will meet people who will help you to make connections with other physicians, or who will open doors for you.

4. Contact the AIMG Program office and stay connected with them. Keep up to date on the next application dates, and be sure that you

are doing everything you need to do to be ready at the next application date.

5. Get involved in the AIMGA. You will get to know other IMGs who are working toward the same goal. You will be able to help each other along the way and you will not feel so alone.

6. Be patient and do not give up your dream. Keep reminding yourself that opportunities are improving for IMGs in Alberta and in Canada.

AUTHOR'S NOTE

On behalf of the research team, I would like to sincerely thank the IMGs who took the time to share their stories. Their dedication and determination to reach their goal sets an example for those who will be involved in making the changes that need to take place to reduce the barriers and increase the supports for IMGs to re-enter medical practice in Alberta and Canada. It is our hope that this collection of stories will help make the IMG journey easier.

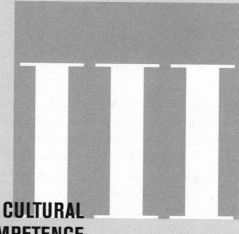

CULTURAL COMPETENCE AND LANGUAGE IN MEDICAL PRACTICE

OVERVIEW

Language is a key element of culture, and communication between patients and health care providers is integral to the provision of quality health services. Effective communication between patients and providers is important for conveying information, establishing a good interpersonal relationship, and making treatment-related decisions. For many immigrants to Canada, language is a barrier to accessing health services. Even when English language proficiency appears to be adequate, cultural differences in the perception, meaning, and communication of health problems can pose challenges to the medical encounter. Language nuances, absence of translation between languages, and differences in the perceptions of the meaning of illness within a cultural context can hinder communication. Not only is language an issue for immigrant patients, but also for immigrant health care providers. In Canada, professional language proficiency for immigrant health care professionals is essential for professional integration into the health care system. Two aspects of communication are explored in this section—the assessment of international medical graduates (IMGs) in English language proficiency and the importance of language in the provision of health care services.

In "Language Proficiency Programs and Professional Integration of International Medical Graduate," David Watt and Deidre Lake explore the difficulties posed by the diverse discourses of IMGs. Not only must IMGs acclimatize themselves to Canadian culture and integrate their families into schools and work environments dramatically different than "home," but they must meet certain criteria in order to practise in Canada. Language proficiency is one of these criteria. While various programs have been developed to speed the language proficiency of immigrant doctors, this chapter specifically examines the Language Communication Assessment Project, whose purpose is to jump-start the integration of immigrant physicians into medical practice. This program has shown considerable success, and the outcomes of its approach are elucidated.

Sparked by clinical experience and collaborative research on cultural diversity, Jean Triscott observed that language was a barrier to accessing health services in the geriatric medical context for certain ethnic/cultural groups. Her chapter "Reflections on Language in the Management of Dementia" explores issues concerning the influence of language on the understanding of disease, second-language difficulties, language reversion, and translation. More research and improved services are needed in the area of the interface of language and the health care system in Canada.

For health care professionals, cultural competence is integral to effective communication with culturally/ethnically diverse patient populations. Cultural perspectives of both patients and health care providers can influence communication, access to and utilization of health services, and patients' perceptions of the care they receive. In "Cultural Competence of Health Professionals," Olga Szafran, Earle Waugh, and Jean Triscott examine the clinical cultural competence of health care providers working in select Cree, francophone, Lebanese Muslim, and Chinese communities in northern Alberta. There is a clear need for health professionals to receive culturally sensitive training.

EIGHT

LANGUAGE PROFICIENCY PROGRAMS AND PROFESSIONAL INTEGRATION OF INTERNATIONAL MEDICAL GRADUATES

David L.E. Watt PhD

Deidre Lake MEd, TESL

BACKGROUND

Immigration has long been recognized as an essential ingredient of Canadian identity, both within Canada and internationally. As a country, we have constantly struggled with the tension between seeing ourselves as a singular, monolithic nation-state and recognizing our reality as an ever-evolving mosaic of cultures and languages (Saul, 1997). Our mosaic, at its simplest, is made up of First Nations people, people who immigrated more than a generation ago, and first-generation immigrants. Our challenge and ultimately our success lies in the degree to which each generation is able to identify and address the emerging social, educational, and occupational integration issues.

The most critical integration issue we face today is the professional integration of skilled immigrants. For the last decade, the national immigration strategy has actively sought to increase the number of skilled immigrants each year. The skilled immigrant category prioritizes individuals with postgraduate levels of education, established professional careers, and high levels of English language proficiency, among other factors (Citizenship and Immigration Canada, 2007). The magnitude of this change in the immigration profile between 1992 and 2004 is most dramatically evident in a single statistic (Picot, Hou, & Coulombe, 2007): 17% of the adult immigrants arriving in 1992 held a university degree; in 2004, university-educated immigrants represented 49% of the annual cohort. It is this single change in the immigration demographic that has brought to public attention the need for each profession to better understand and address its process for the professional integration of immigrants seeking to re-enter their fields and make their contribution to the Canadian mosaic.

The easiest way to capture some of the issues that commonly face immigrant physicians is to contextualize them into a composite narrative, which though fictitious in nature, represents a common story. The relevant details are not extraordinary and easily fit the realities of a large number of IMGS seeking professional reintegration in Canada.

NATASHA'S STORY

Natasha is a 43-year-old physician who was the head of a cardiac surgery team in Moscow. She immigrated to Canada in 2003 as a skilled immigrant and has been trying to re-enter the medical profession ever since. Even though she has passed all the Canadian medical exams required of doctors graduating from Canadian medical schools before their licensure, Natasha still cannot gain direct entry to provincial licensure. The route to licensure requires her to take additional steps. The most notable step is that she must repeat residency training in Canada, and must compete with over 200 other immigrant physicians for one of 49 spots in a 2–5 year residency program. Last year, Natasha was among the 50 per cent of the applicants who successfully met the requirements of the gruelling three-hour examination process. She was required to demonstrate her clinical skills in an extensive set of medical cases where she was evaluated by a team of physician examiners who rated her performance on clinical skills, communication in medical interviews and professional language proficiency. Although Natasha placed in the 95th percentile of candidates in the clinical assessment, a round of interviews designed to reduce the number of candidates to 49 eliminated her from the final assignment of residency positions.

Natasha is determined to find her way into her profession, but she knows that the longer she remains out of practice the more her skills will suffer and her chances of successfully re-entering her field of expertise will be increasingly compromised. So, in order to support her efforts to successfully immigrate and maintain her medical skills, Natasha is obliged to return to Russia for several months every year, where she can practice surgery and earn enough money to continue to pursue the current route for IMGs into Canadian medical practice.

This narrative is far from unique. Many skilled professionals find re-entering their professions to be an exceptionally complicated and difficult process. The resulting underemployment is devastating both in terms of *lost human capital* and *chronic poverty*—two terms coined by Statistics Canada to describe the underemployment of immigrant professionals and the subsequent effect of being trapped in a perpetual low-income cycle.

As Canada increases its focus on highly educated and professional immigrants, the demand for effective programs that advance levels of English language proficiency for professional purposes and assist in the integration of skilled immigrants becomes increasingly evident. Findings from Statistics Canada's second wave of the *Longitudinal Survey of Immigrants to Canada* (Statistics Canada, 2005) found that of the principal applicants in the skilled worker category who were aged 25 to 44, just under half (48%) found a job in their intended occupation. Consider the impact of these results on the 300–500 IMGs presently seeking licensure in Alberta and on a general population that fuels the increasing demand for practising physicians.

According to the Canadian Medical Association, medical schools in Canada are not in a position to produce enough new physicians to meet the demands of a growing population. One commonly reported national strategy relies on the use of International Medical Graduates (IMGs) to augment the physician supply. It has been estimated that approximately 25% of all the practising doctors in Canada are IMGs and further, that IMGs constitute 40% of all the doctors in rural practices (Buske, 1997). While the Canadian Medical Association recognizes the importance of IMGs in its plan for meeting the Canadian physician supply now and in the future, there remains some degree of confusion around the general use of the term IMG. With a few notable exceptions (Nasmith, 1993), the literature related to IMGs and medical practice in Canada does not distinguish between immigrant IMGs and IMGs who are recruited directly from other countries to fill specific positions on either full or provisional provincial licences (Audas, Ross, & Vardy, 2005). In the past, the medical profession has based its reliance more heavily on the availability of "visa doctors." However, today, with the growing numbers of immigrant physicians in Canada, there is a need to balance the two competing strategies for using IMGs in a way that recognizes a national commitment to the professional integration of immigrant physicians. The concern over the backlog of immigrant IMGs seeking professional reintegration is clearly identified in Alberta's immigration plan, which highlights a need to "expand current activities...to attract, license and retain doctors, pharmacists, nurses and other health care professionals" as part of its goal to "remove barriers to immigrants' full participation as equal citizens in all aspects of community life" (Alberta, 2005, p. 10).

MEASUREMENT OF KNOWLEDGE, SKILLS, AND PROFESSIONAL LANGUAGE PROFICIENCY

Notwithstanding the advocacy issues that underlie the professional integration of immigrant physicians, there is the non-trivial issue of establishing appropriate standards that will maximize accessibility while accurately identifying expected standards of Canadian practice. Accountable professional integration through licensure in any profession requires the accurate measurement of expected thresholds in three areas: professional knowledge, professional skill, and professional language proficiency. Nationally, medical knowledge is assessed through the Medical Council of Canada's Evaluating Exam, and Qualifying Exam Part I, where candidates are able to demonstrate the degree to which they meet the basic medical knowledge standard. Their clinical medical skills, related to real-time problem-solving and patient interactions are later assessed through the Qualifying Exam Part II. The specific needs related to assessing the professional readiness of IMG physicians saw the advent of a third measure: a clinical skills assessment that includes thresholds for medical communication and professional language proficiency.

Since 2001, IMGs in Alberta seeking licensure apply through the Alberta International Medical Graduate Program to gain access to the Objective Structured Clinical Examination (OSCE) assessment, where clinical skills, medical communication, and language proficiency are assessed. During this time, one trend has become very clear: the level of professional language proficiency directly affects IMGs' ability to demonstrate their level of clinical skill in the simulated doctor–patient scenarios that constitute the OSCE. There is a general assumption that, if a candidate's professional language proficiency is below the expected threshold, the candidate will not be able to demonstrate his or her skills fully and is not ready to meet the expectations of patients and colleagues in professional practice. It seems simple enough to accept that professional language proficiency for the practice of medicine is essential in determining success in the process of immigrant professional integration. However, the idea that professional language proficiency represents a distinct perspective on the use of language is a new advancement in understanding IMG professional integration.

LANGUAGE: KNOWLEDGE, SKILL, AND PROFICIENCY

Language can be seen as having three distinct aspects: knowledge of the grammatical rules and vocabulary, the skills required to use that knowledge in encoding and decoding messages, and the proficiency to use the knowledge and skills in real-time, unpredictable exchanges with others in order to successfully and strategically accomplish tasks in a manner that is considered acceptable to others. On the one hand, language can be seen as code—a set of rules and patterns; on the other hand, language can be seen as behaviour—the subtle and audience-sensitive manner in which language is used to negotiate meaning in a specific context (Halliday, 1978). Even with an advanced knowledge of a second language and the academic skills associated with reading and writing complex texts, multilingual professionals often show less advanced proficiency in meeting the culturally specific expectations of professional communication.

UNDERSTANDING ENGLISH LANGUAGE PROFICIENCY FOR PROFESSIONAL PURPOSES

A valuable distinction may be drawn between professional language proficiency and other forms of language proficiency. This distinction helps us understand that there is a fundamental difference between the language proficiency needed to learn a discipline like medicine and the kind of proficiency needed to practise that discipline once learned. Professional language proficiency represents the ability to meet the communication demands specific to the roles, responsibilities, and communication tasks of the profession, as judged by members of the profession. This proficiency is distinct from medical language proficiency, the ability to use medical terminology in the discipline of medicine. Medical language proficiency is a subset of academic language proficiency, which is most often associated with the ability to study and communicate within an academic discipline. Academic language proficiency is distinct from general language proficiency, which represents the ability to carry out communication successfully in the kinds of daily interactions that are more common to the general population. While there are commonalities among the different proficiencies, they are not necessarily identical. Professional expectations around appropriate communication are culturally specific. There are subtle norms around how to elicit a patient's medical history, inquire into sensitive personal issues, negotiate a management and treatment plan, and break bad news in a patient-centred approach to the practice of medicine. For example, a clinically competent doctor from a different medical tradition may have a very different style of interacting and communicating with colleagues and patients than what would be expected in the cultural practice of medicine in Canada. Adjusting to these cultural differences brings with it new language demands and the need to become proficient in communicating in a manner that meets the cultural expectations of colleagues and patients.

When IMGs apply for immigration as skilled immigrants, they undergo an assessment of general language proficiency as part of their application. They are awarded points for English language proficiency based on performance on TOEFL (Test of English as a Foreign Language), IELTS (International English Language Testing System), or CLB (Canadian Language Benchmarks). On the CLB, candidates usually achieve benchmarks in the range of CLB 6–8:

Benchmark 6

Can comprehend and relate audio-mediated information. Understands and uses a wide variety of sentence structures. Discourse is reasonably fluent. Grammar and pronunciation errors may sometimes impede communication. Comprehends and uses a range of common and idiomatic language.

Benchmark 7

Can discuss concrete information on a familiar topic. Comfortably engages in a conversation at a descriptive level. Discourse is fluent.

Grammar and pronunciation errors rarely impede communication. Uses an expanded inventory of concrete and idiomatic language.

Benchmark 8
Can comprehend and synthesize abstract ideas on a familiar topic. Comfortably engages in a conversation at an abstract level. Discourse is fluent. Grammar and pronunciation errors do not impede communication. Uses an expanded inventory of concrete, idiomatic and conceptual language. (Pawlikowska-Smith, 2000)

While these descriptors denote a reasonably advanced level of general proficiency, typically there is a gap between these levels and the specific demands on language that relate to professional communication. The general assumption is that either time or direct instruction will be needed to raise language proficiency to the levels expected for professional practice (i.e., a range generally between CLB 8 and CLB 10).

Previous studies have been able to establish approximate rates of acquisition for general language proficiency. In a recent Canadian study (Watt & Lake, 2004) of adult immigrant language learners enrolled in language instruction classes, a rate for each benchmark of language growth was calculated in terms of direct hours of language instruction. For individuals with 17+ years of education (i.e., professional immigrants), who were at a CLB 6 and needed to achieve a CLB of 8 to be considered ready for professional examination processes in fields like medicine, the average length of time was calculated at 880 hours of instruction, or approximately one year of full-time study. Even after achieving CLB 8 in general language proficiency, professional immigrants usually need to attune their proficiency to the demands of professional communication.

The recognition of the time required to achieve English language proficiency is a critical element in understanding the path of professional reintegration. There is a general consensus in the medical profession that the length of time a physician is out of practice adversely affects the chances of successful reintegration, and in some jurisdictions an absence of more than five years is considered to jeopardize safe and competent practice (Recency of Practice Requirements). This phenomenon sometimes referred to as the recency effect, increases the urgency of identifying at-risk immigrant IMGs and providing suitable language training programs to minimize the delay in reaching professional readiness. It also underscores two valuable insights: general language proficiency does not necessarily lead to similar levels of professional language proficiency, and language instruction for general language proficiency may not suffice for attaining professional language proficiency in a new culture.

LANGUAGE, CULTURE, AND MEDICAL CULTURE

Each language and culture has unwritten rules about the degree of clarity, brevity, truth, and relevance expected in the communication of ideas. These conversational maxims of communication and their implicature (Grice, 1975) are learned through experience. The degree of directness or indirectness of a person's speech (Searle, 1990) can make it difficult to interpret the meaning behind what is said, even with a fairly refined understanding of the language itself. Getting the degree of directness wrong can cause communication to be interpreted as too abrupt or too wordy, too pointed or too obscure, uncaringly truthful or unrevealing, irrelevant or underexplained. The act of communicating in a first or second language, in real time and for a real purpose, is always susceptible to subtle and unintentional cues that are sometimes misinterpreted and can relay accidental messages (Saville-Troike, 2003) about the speaker's attitude or the perceived importance of what is said. With second-language speakers, there is an increased risk that unintended accidental messages will cause the communication to be misinterpreted or derailed, and eventually break down. The way ideas are expressed, the way language is used to signal interpersonal relations, the way people physically position themselves (Hall, 1966), and even the voice quality and intonation patterns (Watt, 1992) used by a speaker can significantly affect how a listener interprets a speaker's meaning. The primary source of these communication breakdowns is not in the meaning of what is said, but in the manner in which it is relayed. The subtleties of how something is expressed are culturally determined through our experience with language as behaviour, not language as code. In order to learn these subtleties, second-language speakers need the opportunity to gain experience in communicating in relevant situations and adjusting their performance to meet the expected norms of language as behaviour (Halliday, 1984).

The impact of culture on communication has been well documented and is often visible in even the shortest and simplest of exchanges between people. Cultural expectations about the meaning of actions, events, relations, and expressions are the residue of the life experiences that make up small-c culture. Small-c culture has been described as the sum of the generic situations that constitute the life experience of an individual. Looked at from this perspective, cultural competence is the by-product of a person's experience in interacting with others in the types of situations that commonly occur. For example, there are common beliefs, assumptions, and practices that relate to situations like buying a car, interviewing for a job, visiting the dentist, or attending a parent–teacher interview. Individuals develop their understanding of how each situation should proceed, what their role is, and what is considered appropriate in the interaction. Similarities and differences across cultures can be seen in the degree to which generic situations and their expectations compare.

Professional culture and, more specifically, medical culture also differ from country to country. The differences are evident in such areas as:

- the approach to medical practice (doctor-centred vs. patient-centred care)
- the preferences in clinical management plans (crutches vs. walkers)
- the commonality and frequency of reported illness (depression vs. infection)
- health care system and available support services (home care vs. social services).

In the cultural practice of doctor-centred medicine, the interaction between doctors and patients is quite different from the patient-centred approach. The language used to achieve the expected communication in one approach is insufficient for meeting the expectations of the other. Often, the source of perceived language difficulties lies in an IMG's lack of familiarity with the culturally appropriate responses expected by patients in the practice of patient-centred medicine. Cultures also differ regarding clinical management plans, often as a result of prevailing practice or availability of supplies. One simple example of the adverse effect of this difference in the assessment of medical competence was made visible in the development of the Australian Occupational English Test (2007) for immigrant physicians, where mismatches in preferred uses of walkers and crutches led to negative interpretations of the quality of medical practice. IMGs themselves have noted that the frequency of commonly reported illnesses differs from country to country and that their professional responses to the different cases may be less developed in some areas in which they are less familiar (i.e., depression). Lastly, the various support services available in the Canadian medical culture adds another element that can affect how a doctor responds to a patient's needs.

Slight differences in both common culture and medical culture affect how a doctor addresses a patient, inquires about a patient's medical history, explains diagnoses, and suggests management plans. By focusing an IMG's learning on the language used in the communication and interpretation of doctor–patient exchanges in generic medical situations, it is possible to develop and assess an IMG's proficiency in meeting the communication expectations of Canadian medical practice. In order to demonstrate their ability to meet these expectations, IMGs must undergo an assessment process, which is itself embedded with cultural expectations.

THE ROLE OF AUTHENTIC ASSESSMENT OF PROFESSIONAL LANGUAGE PROFICIENCY

Internationally, the most significant advancement in the assessment of language for professional purposes has been the move toward authentic assessment. Authentic assessment is the assessment of language proficiency in situations and tasks that are specific to the profession (Douglas, 2000). The closer these tasks are to the real-world expectations of the profession, the more accurately they can predict performance in the field.

The goal of authentic assessment is to simulate the conditions of professional interaction. Such assessments need to accurately sample the range of experiences that are most likely to be representative of the communication demands of professional practice. While not identical to genuine experiences, the interaction requires test takers to engage strategically in solving unpredictable problems by communicating in real time. It is in the quality of the interaction that holistic and analytic decisions can be made about the language proficiency evidenced in the performance of the task and thresholds can be established that reflect the judgements of both medical colleagues and standardized patients (SPs), in an effort to predict the likely communication success of future professional interactions.

Assessments such as these typically employ both holistic and analytic rating scales (Douglas, 2000). Holistic assessments often include questions similar to the following:

• Did the candidate successfully complete the task in an appropriate manner?

- Did the candidate demonstrate sufficient language proficiency to be my colleague?
- Did the candidate demonstrate sufficient language proficiency to be my doctor?

Analytic criteria further break down the holistic reactions into categories related to fluency, pronunciation, comprehensibility, vocabulary, and grammar. The use of mixed-rating scales is widely supported in the international literature on authentic assessment for professional language proficiency. On the one hand, holistic decisions allow practitioners to express their general reactions; on the other hand, analytic decisions help refine the discussion of the holistic reactions.

An examination process like the OSCE is exceptionally well positioned to meet the requirements for the authentic assessment of professional language proficiency. It uses multiple cases and examiners, authentic tasks, real-time communication, and a rating scale that has been adapted from the national standard CLB scales to reflect medical contexts, based on the authors' observations of IMGs in the OSCE. These observations were the impetus behind the Language Communication Assessment Project (L-CAP). It was clear that some candidates were struggling to communicate and to conduct a medical interview in a manner that was considered appropriate for a Canadian context. It is clear that IMGs find that performance-based exams challenge their understanding of the cultural and communication demands. Instruction, exposure, and feedback are necessary in order for IMGs to apply their medical knowledge and skills successfully within a Canadian medical context. While it seems obvious to point out that the cultural expectations around acceptable medical communication are learned through experience and over time, the question remains whether it is possible to accelerate the learning of professional language proficiency through an instructional style that would help immigrant physicians understand the nuances associated with communicating their clinical skills.

THE LANGUAGE COMMUNICATION ASSESSMENT PROJECT

The aim of the L-CAP program was to prepare recent immigrant physicians to meet the communication and language requirements associated with Canadian medical practice. The program sought to accelerate the rate at which IMGs could develop their professional language proficiency through a performance-based teaching approach. The approach involves

professional actors, medical cases, videotaped coaching, language instructors, and assessors. The premise of the approach was that by increasing
professional language proficiency, IMGs would be more able to demonstrate the scope of their clinical medical skills (Friedman, Sutnick, Stillman,
Regan, & Nocini, 1993). The expected result would be an increased chance
of success in moving forward to medical residency and then on to medical
practice. The program took place in the Faculty of Medicine at the University of Calgary, in association with the Alberta Immigrant Medical Graduate
Program. It consisted of two major components: an intensive eight-week
instructional component, and an instructionally supported eight-week clinical work placement.

The Participants

The 25 participants selected from across Alberta had all successfully completed the required medical knowledge exams—the Medical Council of
Canada Evaluating Exam and the subsequent Qualifying Exam Part I. The
participants represented a wide range of countries of origin, languages, and
medical expertise. They were selected based on a level of English language
proficiency that was advanced but not sufficient for successful medical
practice. The Canadian Language Benchmarks Assessment was used to
select IMGs who met or exceeded the following language profile: listening/
speaking CLB 7, reading CLB 8, writing CLB 7. More than half the participants
had been unsuccessful at the next medical examination stage (the OSCE),
which offers access to a limited number of residency positions for IMGs.
Their goals were to pass the OSCE and move forward to residency. Of the 24
IMGs who completed the L-CAP program, all either were landed immigrants
(61.9%) or Canadian citizens (38.1%). They were on average 40 years of age,
and had lived in Canada for about 4.5 years (see table 1).

Program Goals

The L-CAP program sought to address the goal of advancing professional
integration and language proficiency through the following actions:

1. Develop a language training program for immigrant IMGs who
    were permanent residents or Canadian citizens of Alberta, had
    advanced levels of English language proficiency (listening/speak-
    ing CLB 7, reading CLB 8, writing CLB 7 or higher), had graduated
    from an institution recognized by the World Health Organization,

TABLE 1: *Participant Demographics in the Language Communication Assessment Project*

IMG Characteristic		IMGs
Sex	Female	57.1%
	Male	42.9%
Age	30–39	42.9%
	40–49	52.3%
	50	4.8%
	Mean age	39.48
Country	Afghanistan	1
	Brazil	1
	Bulgaria	1
	China	3
	Columbia	3
	India	3
	Nigeria	1
	Pakistan	6
	Philippines	1
	Russia	2
	Sri Lanka	1
	Ukraine	2
First Language	Bulgarian	1
	Chinese	3
	Farsi	1
	Hiligaynon	1
	Ibo	1
	Portuguese	1
	Punjabi	2
	Russian	2
	Sinhalese	1
	Spanish	3
	Telugu	1
	Ukrainian	2
	Urdu	6
Immigrant Status	Canadian citizen	38.1%
	Landed immigrant	61.9%
Years in Canada	1–2	24.0%
	2.1–4	32.0%
	4.1–6	20.0%
	6.1+	24.0%
	Mean years	4.50
Employment status at project start	Employed full-time	30.4%
	Employed part-time	26.1%
	Unemployed, seeking work	21.7%
	Unemployed, not seeking work	17.4%
	Student	4.3%
Total N		25

and had successfully completed the Medical Council of Canada Evaluating Exam.

2. Develop strong professional ties by locating the program inside the Health Sciences building at the University of Calgary for access to medical libraries and the MedSkills Centre, by involving doctors and health regions, and by insuring that participants obtained courtesy licences for their eight-week clinical placement and approval from health regions where applicable.

3. Create a program structure aimed at professional language proficiency by focusing on a structured performance-based curricular approach to language development, using SPs (actors playing standardized patients) and simulated medical cases, and by including both classroom instruction and workplace experience and instruction.

4. Create a curriculum aimed at preparation for communication in Canadian medical practice by introducing the cultural component of patient-centred care, using the Calgary-Cambridge Guide to the Medical Interview–Communication Process (an established set of process skills for successful physician–patient interviews [GP-training.net, 2006]), using medical professionals in the selection of relevant medical communication cases, and sequencing medical communication cases in order of increasing language difficulty.

5. Enhance the quality of feedback by videotaping individual performances twice each week and by using language assessment experts and medical experts in the weekly participant feedback cycles.

6. Track the rate and growth of professional language proficiency by using repeated measures of the Canadian Language Benchmarks Assessment, and the CLB-compatible OSCE language proficiency assessment results.

7. Track the outcomes: the number of candidates who successfully passed the OSCE and the number of candidates who successfully took up residency seats or other professional employment in medicine.

8. Weekly validation of the program's results through direct feedback from professionals in the field and by undergoing an external

evaluation of the program and its delivery by a government-recognized evaluation consultant.

9. Engage in ongoing research to advance the professional integration process for immigrant IMGs by clearing University of Calgary ethics approval for the development of video tools based on participant performances and language acquisition data and by developing new models for the development and assessment of professional language proficiency in medicine that can be applied across provincial jurisdictions.

Program Design

The L-CAP program was designed around a unique, performance-based curriculum approach to the development of English for professional practice. It uses language teachers, standardized clinical case scenarios, physician feedback, and SPs to create authentic and dynamic communication situations relevant to the practice of family medicine. The program delivery followed a weekly template of in-class preparation activities, coached role-plays, individual videotaped performances on rehearsed medical cases, daily feedback and reflection, and a final videotaped performance for each participant on unrehearsed medical cases, organized in a hierarchy of increasing communicative complexity. The curriculum was organized around "Week-at-a-Glance" curricular templates, which integrated the learning objectives with the clinical case objectives, the professional language functions as specified by the Calgary-Cambridge Guide to the Medical Interview–Communication Process framework, and the language assessment and individual observations. The program was intent on measuring four specific outcomes:

- The improvement in language proficiency using a performance-based approach
- The gains in clinical performance that may result from better communication skills
- The participants' perceptions of readiness for Canadian medical practice after L-CAP
- The concrete results of success in attaining a residency position for L-CAP participants.

PERFORMANCE-BASED CURRICULUM

There are a variety of ways of organizing curricula for language-teaching goals. For the purposes of advancing the professional language proficiency for individuals that already have a great deal of general language proficiency (i.e., CLB 7 or higher), the candidate's challenge is to make micro-adjustments that more accurately reflect the expectations of communicating with patients. These micro-adjustments to the way things are said and the way conversations are negotiated can be most effectively addressed using a performance-based curriculum model. The performance-based model permits for direct, individual feedback in repeated practice situations as participants internalize the expected language performance on relevant medical interactions. Where performance-based curriculum differs from other curricular approaches is in the priority placed on language as behaviour and the importance given to immediate feedback to the development of language proficiency for specific purposes. In order to internalize language as behaviour, it is practised in a variety of controlled role-plays, rehearsed live cases, and unrehearsed live cases, with structured feedback on each candidate's performance and specific advice for how to improve each exchange with the simulated patient.

THE ROLE OF STRUCTURED FEEDBACK

Feedback differs from testing and assessment in significant ways. The feedback is ongoing and immediate. It can provide individuals with accurate and clear information that they use as the impetus for either clinical (Hewson & Little, 1998) or language and communication (Roter et al., 2004) change. Feedback can be given on aspects as discreet as voice quality, wording, gestures and body language; or it can address holistic matters such as cultural nuances, unintended meanings, and the interpretation of interpersonal relations. Feedback differs at different points along the continuum of instruction and learning. Feedback varies in type as the rehearsal of performances becomes increasingly authentic (i.e., from group setting to role-play scenarios in class, to rehearsed cases with SPs, to unrehearsed cases with SPs, to clinics with real patients). As learners move themselves forward toward authentic interaction with simulated patients who respond in unexpected ways, feedback in the form of coaching and critique is used to move learners from supported, predictable contexts to independent, unpredictable contexts. Structured feedback from dependent to independent contexts provides one critical aspect; the other critical aspect of feedback is the use of multiple perspectives.

For feedback to be fully effective, not only must instructors, peers, and SPs provide their observations, but also the individual needs the opportunity to review his or her own performances and critique them in light of others' feedback. By using videotape as a primary teaching tool, it is possible to provide direct feedback about each individual's professional interaction and, as a result, to accelerate the rate of change in the full range of communication related cues, from body language and voice quality to speech functions and doctor–patient exchanges.

The balance of performance-based curriculum and feedback was considered the most effective way to accelerate change and to familiarize IMGs with the cultural and language expectations of Canadian medical practice.

THE ROLE OF INSTRUCTIONAL METHODOLOGY

Instruction in a performance-based model must also be distinct to be effective. Rather than focusing on content or the development of language knowledge, instruction is directly related to the language performance of learners as they move through unscripted medical cases of increasing communicative difficulty. Instructors in a performance-based model are more like film directors than facilitators. They are responsible for providing learners with specific directions to follow, clear expectations, and a constructive critique of performance. Therefore, the instructional techniques are focused on building capacity and moving individuals through a hierarchy of rehearsed performances; then a critique of unrehearsed performances develops the capacity for change in performance and professional proficiency.

Instructional methodology in a performance-based curriculum relies on the resilience of its participants: they must be willing to accept and act on constructive feedback. IMGs are highly educated, have an advanced level of general language proficiency, and are determined to meet the standards required for licensure in Canada. The instructional methodology also places demand on instructors, who must be capable of providing direct, relevant, and instantaneous feedback to participants in order to direct change. The change must be visible to the learners themselves and lead to positive improvement in a performance of unrehearsed, timed, medical interviews.

THE ROLE OF WORKPLACE EXPERIENCE

The role of the workplace experience is an integral element of any English Language Training (ELT) program, a federally funded language initiative for immigrant professionals. It is the ultimate proving ground for the development of professional language proficiency. It provides participants with the least supported, least predictable, most independent context for the practice of their clinical and communication skills in a Canadian context. It allows them to see the relevance of the changes they have made and the understanding they have gained in patient-centred communication and care.

The workplace requires physicians who are willing to act as mentors and to assist and evaluate change. An instructional component where participants have a place to discuss the challenges they face and continue to learn from one another is an essential component in the success of participants' integration into the Canadian medical profession.

It is the combination of these components that affords participants the opportunity to demonstrate their medical knowledge, clinical skills, and language proficiency for professional purposes within an assessment.

THE OUTCOMES

The following sections outline the measurable results for the four intended outcomes of the program: language gains, clinical gains, participant perceptions, and concrete outcomes. Each outcome addresses a major issue in the advocacy-oriented goals of demonstrating the viability of enhancing immigrant physician readiness for professional integration.

The First Outcome: Language Gains

Table 2 presents the increase in English language proficiency from the onset of the program to the end of the practicum placement. It demonstrates the growth in general language proficiency that occurred over the duration of the program and its 200 hours of direct instruction. Despite the ceiling effect that is created by approaching the upper bound (CLB 8) of the test, L-CAP participants demonstrated a statistically significant gain (p<.01) of a half benchmark in speaking and listening, as well as in writing.

The L-CAP participants exceeded the general rate of language acquisition that has been established for professionals with a similar educational background and a similar level of English language proficiency (Watt & Lake, 2004). L-CAP participants improved at a rate 30% faster than the

TABLE 2: *Language Proficiency Gains Pre/Post* L-CAP

Skill Area	Mean Benchmark Level			Statistical Test
	Before L-CAP	After L-CAP	Mean Gain	
Listening/speaking	7.17	7.61	.44	t = 4.1, df = 22, p<.01
Reading	7.91	7.96	.05	t = 1.0, df = 22, p>.30
Writing	6.91	7.43	.52	t = 3.8, df = 22, p<.01

comparison group. The total language proficiency gain was calculated after the completion of the OSCE exam. Each is represented in table 3, which demonstrates a total mean gain of 1.12 benchmarks in speaking and listening and 1.89 benchmarks in writing in medical contexts.

TABLE 3: *Participants' Language Benchmark Gain after* L-CAP

Skill Area	Mean Benchmark Level			Statistical Test
	Before L-CAP	OSCE 2006	Mean Gain	
Listening/speaking	7.24	8.36	1.12	t = 7.7, df = 20, p<.001
Writing	6.90	8.36	1.89	t = 9.8, df = 2-, p<.001

The Second Outcome: Clinical Gains

The L-CAP program increased the participants' ability to demonstrate their existing clinical skills through a measured change in their professional language proficiency. For the L-CAP participants who had taken the OSCE exam before, only 47% had met the Minimum Proficiency Level prior to L-CAP. Over 73% met the threshold clinical score after L-CAP. The average gain of approximately 10% in the OSCE scores was noted as impressive by the external evaluator. Furthermore, 93% of the participants improved their overall score. The average scores for each component of the exam are presented in table 4. The gains are statistically significant.

TABLE 4: *Participants' Increase in* OSCE *Scores after* L-CAP

OSCE Sub-Scores	Mean Level			Statistical Test
	Before L-CAP	After L-CAP	Percentage Point Gain	
Overall	61.61%	71.65%	10.04%	t = 6.1, df = 14, p<.001
Clinical	58.61%	69.18%	10.57%	t = 5.8, df = 14, p<.001
Communication	66.89%	76.78%	9.89%	t = 5.2, df = 14, p<.001
Language	65.34%	72.47%	7.13%	t = 4.3, df = 13, p<.001
Writing	—	87.86%	—	

The Third Outcome: Participant Perceptions

Readiness and confidence are two critical factors for professional integration. The longer it takes to return to practice, the less prepared and the less confident physicians become. Figures 1 and 2 demonstrate that the L-CAP program advanced the participants' sense of understanding of the Canadian medical system and was effective in redressing the lack of confidence that may have accrued from the participants' previous unsuccessful experiences with professional integration.

Figure 1: Extent to Which L-CAP Participation Increased Confidence

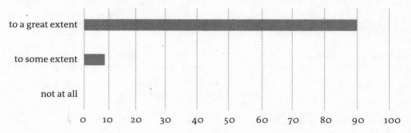

Figure 2: Extent to Which L-CAP Participation Increased Understanding

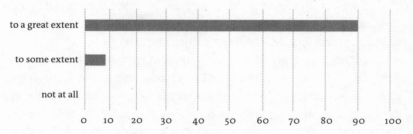

The Fourth Outcome: Concrete Results

Of the 24 participants in the pilot project, 20 chose to enrol in the OSCE. From this group, 14 met the OSCE examination thresholds and were selected to advance to the interviewing stage. Of the 14, 10 were selected for the 49 available residency seats in Alberta, and one took a residency position in the United States. In total, 11 L-CAP participants obtained residency seats, and 4 participants obtained clinical assistant positions. Clinical assistant positions are paid positions that provide IMGs with the opportunity to practise under the supervision of an attending physician, while expanding their Canadian medical experience prior to retaking the OSCE. In short, 50% of the L-CAP participants gained access to residency programs and another 20% were able to advance their professional status by taking up clinical assistant positions. This success rate compares favourably to the general success rate for attaining residency through the OSCE, where the rate is 49 out of 198 or approximately 25%.

CONCLUSION

The measurable successes of the L-CAP program in forwarding the professional integration of immigrant IMGs helps to demonstrate the important role that instructional programs can play in the process. It underscores a need to distinguish between the use of non-resident IMGs to fill needed short-term positions in the physician supply and our national responsibility to support and advocate for the long-term professional integration of immigrant IMGs. Existing examination processes like the OSCE offer an accountable way of measuring the clinical skills, medical communication, and professional language proficiency deemed necessary for professional integration. Professional language proficiency appears to play a critical role in an IMG's capacity to accurately demonstrate the degree of clinical skills required for professional integration. The development of language proficiency and, more specifically, professional language proficiency requires direct experience with the expectations of professional communication in the practice of medicine. Given the urgency to re-enter the profession as quickly as possible in order to avoid the deterioration of skills, an instructional program based on structured cases that present a broad range of communication situations can act as a means of accelerating the growth of professional language proficiency and the capacity to demonstrate professional readiness. Professional language proficiency is rooted in an understanding of the cultural expectations around doctor–patient communication, and a program like the L-CAP program can positively affect the development of an IMG's ability to interpret and communicate effectively in the culturally determined practice of medicine in Canada.

REFERENCES

Alberta. (2005, July 15). *Supporting immigrants and immigration to Alberta.* Edmonton: Human Resources and Employment. Accessed November 28, 2007, from Alberta Employment and Immigration website: http://employment. alberta.ca/documents/ WIA/WIA-IM_policy_framework.pdf

Audas, R., Ross, A., & Vardy, D. (2005). The use of provisionally licensed international medical graduates in Canada. *Canadian Medical Association Journal, 173(11)*, 1315–16.

Buske, L. (1997). Canada's international medical graduates. *Canadian Medical Association Journal, 157(1)*, 116.

Citizenship and Immigration Canada. (2007). Skilled workers and professionals. Accessed November 28, 2007, at http://www.cic.gc.ca/english/immigrate/skilled/index.asp

Douglas, D. (2000). *Assessing languages for specific purposes.* Cambridge: Cambridge University Press.

Friedman, M., Sutnick, A., Stillman, P., Regan, M., & Nocini, J. (1993). The relationship of Sken-English proficiencies of foreign medical graduates to their clinical competence. *Academic Medicine, 68(10)*, S1–S3.

GP-training.net. (2006). Calgary-Cambridge guide to the medical interview–communication process. Accessed June 7, 2010, at http://www.gp-training.net/training/communication_skills/calgary/guide.htm

Grice, H.P. (1975). Logic and conversation. In P. Cole & J. Morgan (Eds.), *Syntax and semantics: Speech acts* (vol. 3, pp. 41–58). New York: Academic Press.

Hall, E.T. (1966). *The hidden dimension.* Garden City, NY: Doubleday.

Halliday, M.A.K. (1978). *Language as a social semiotic: The social interpretation of language and meaning.* Baltimore, MD: University Park Press; London: Edward Arnold.

————. (1984). *The semiotics of culture and language.* London: Pinter.

Healy, J.M., Maffi, C.L., & Dugdale, P. (2008). A national medical register: Balancing public transparency and professional privacy. *Medical Journal of Australia, 188(4)*, 247–49. Accessed June 20, 2010, at http://www.mja.com.au/public/issues/188_04_180208/hea10243_fm.pdf

Hewson, M.G., & Little, M.L. (1998). Giving feedback in medical education: Verification of recommended techniques. *Journal of General Internal Medicine, 13(2)*, 111–16.

Nasmith, L. (1993). Programs for international medical graduates. *Canadian Family Physician, 39*, 2549–53.

Pawlikowska-Smith, G. *Canadian Language Benchmarks 2000: English as a second language—for adults.* 54. Accessed September 15, 2010, at http://www.language.ca/pdfs/clb_adults.pdf

Picot, G., Hou, F., & Coulombe, S. (2007). *Chronic low income and low-income dynamics among recent immigrants* (catalogue no. 11 F0019MIE-No.294). Ottawa: Statistics Canada. Accessed November 28, 2007, at http://www.statcan.ca/english/research/11F0019MIE/11F0019MIE2007294.htm

Saul, J.R. (1997). *Reflections of a siamese twin: Canada at the end of the twentieth century.* Toronto: Penguin.

Roter, D.L., Lawson, S., Shinitzky, H., Chernoff, R., Serwint, J.R., Adamo, G., & Wissow, L. (2004). Use of an innovative video feedback technique to enhance communication skills training. *Medical Education, 38(2)*, 145–57.

Saville-Troike, M. (2003). *The ethnography of communication: An introduction* (3rd ed.). London: Blackwell.

Searle, J. (1990). Collective intentions and actions. In M.P.R. Cohen & M. and E. Pollack (Eds.), *Intentions in communication* (pp. 401–16). Cambridge, MA: MIT Press.

Statistics Canada. (2005). *Longitudinal Survey of Immigrants to Canada: A Portrait of Early Settlement Experiences.* Ottawa: Queen's Printer. Accessed November 28, 2007, from Depository Services Program, Government of Canada website: http://dsp-psd.communication.gc.ca/Collection/Statcan/89-614-XIE/89-614-XIE.html

Watt, D.L.E. (1992). *The phonology and semology of intonation in English: An instrumental analysis.* Bloomington: Indiana University Linguistic Club Press.

Watt, D., & Lake, D. (2004). *Benchmarking adult rates of second language acquisition and integration: How long and how fast? Final Report.* Accessed November 28, 2007, from Centre for Canadian Language Benchmarks website: http://www.language.ca/pdfs/Benchmarking%20Adult%20Rates%20of%20Second%20Language%20Acquisition%20and%20Integration1.pdf

NINE

REFLECTIONS ON LANGUAGE IN THE MANAGEMENT OF DEMENTIA

Jean A.C. Triscott MD, CCFP, FCFP

BACKGROUND

In my capacity as geriatric physician in the Memory Clinic for northern Alberta, Canada, I had limited referrals to the clinic from ethnic communities. This is surprising, since ethnic diversity continues to be the norm in the province. In my experience, ethnic patients and their families commonly access resources of the health services system only in the late stages of the dementia, almost beyond the point of effective care. This often results in family crises and ineffective care. Then health care professionals must interact with the family and community during a very stressful time, usually with limited success.

My own experience and informal consultation with colleagues and others have made it evident that both culture and language were playing a key role in the health of several geriatric cases in ethnic communities. Obviously, it was important to determine just how these might be affecting health care practice with my geriatric patients, and especially those with signs of dementia. This information was further necessary for my early diagnosis of this disease, when I could be of most help to my patients. Since I was seeing these patients when they were well on in the disease, I was much less able to help them and their families. It was also crucial to understand how the cultures of these different patients regarded dementia (e.g., whether it *was* considered a disease), since the attitudes toward it were mixed and sometimes families treated my diagnosis with great reserve.

With regard to language, sometimes I relied on interpreters to convey information to my patients, and it soon became evident that interpreters were influencing communication in critical ways. Indeed, there was evidence that interpreters were influencing both the basic information and the medical diagnosis in ways unknown to me or other physicians and health care professionals. Similarly, it seemed significant to me and my colleagues that language skills greatly influenced communication between caregivers (i.e., families) and the health care professions in the later stage of the disease, particularly regarding what could be done to assist with caregiving. Since we were not quite sure what had been said, we were not clear that the caregivers knew what they could face as the disease progressed. Based on our experience in the Memory Clinic environment, it was obvious that effective diagnosis and management of patients, as well as the response of their families, were being impacted by cultural and linguistic factors. It was our research on dementia in five communities that alerted me to the many dimensions of this conclusion.

MEDICAL LITERATURE ON DEMENTIA AND CULTURAL FACTORS

While it could be argued that research on topics directly related to our clinical experience was limited, the main parameters of dementia *as a disease* are well-known. Much work has been accomplished on establishing the foundations of various dementias. Dementia is a diagnosis that refers to a group of progressive neurological disorders characterized by acquired, persistent, and multiple impairments in memory and other cognitive abilities that interfere with a patient's usual social or occupational functioning (American Psychiatric Association, 1994). Furthermore, dementia is a major public health problem and its relevance will increase even further in the upcoming years because both prevalence and incidence are on the rise. The prevalence of dementia doubles with every five years of increase in patients' age, and this rate will increase by 50% during the next 25 years without major advances in prevention (Hofman et al., 1991; Ernst & Hay, 1994). The prevalence of dementia and depression among elders from several ethnic minority groups in the United Kingdom is generally similar to or higher than that among Indigenous elders in Canada (Bhatnagar & Frank, 1997; Lindesay, Jagger, Hibbett, Peet, & Moledina, 1997a; McCracken et al., 1997; Livingston et al., 2001).

Ethnicity and Alzheimer's Disease

It is the case, however, that issues of ethnicity and culture, as they relate to Alzheimer's disease and related disorders, continue to be understudied. Across three ethnic groups in Mahoney, Clouterbuck, Neary, and Zhan's (2005) meta-synthesis of three qualitative studies, there were striking similarities in the reported lack of knowledge about early signs of Alzheimer's disease. Informants attributed initial impressions of an elderly relative's loss of memory to "normal" aging and thus did not deem the memory loss important. All participants conveyed striking similarities of thought about normalization of cognitive symptoms until one critical event, usually relocation, precipitated family awareness that an elder's behaviour was the result of more than normal aging. In this study, a lack of knowledge about Alzheimer's disease, rather than culturally influenced beliefs, was the major deterrent to having an elder's memory assessed. However, stigmatization of persons with Alzheimer's disease was noted among some Chinese patients. Where ethno-cultural differences were noted, there were many similarities in needs that offer health care providers an opportunity to improve quality of care in Alzheimer's disease outreach, education, and professionals' services. Mahoney et al. (2005) suggest providing the public with more confidential access to Alzheimer's disease information, increasing dementia awareness among community physicians, motivating clinicians to adopt culturally sensitive communication patterns, and providing community education to reduce normalization by families and stigmatization of persons with Alzheimer's disease.

Culture, Diagnosis, and Stigmatization

Other research has indicated that cultural values and beliefs about illness and disease among different ethnic groups could shape the meanings assigned to dementia (Dilworth-Anderson & Gibson, 2002). These values and beliefs extended to who gave care and why, as well as whether caregivers sought help outside the family system. Thus, depending on the particular cultural group, the behaviours of a demented older person might not be brought to the attention of medical professionals; instead, these behaviours may be normalized or self-treated by these groups (Chrisman & Kleinman, 1983; Dilworth-Anderson & Anderson, 1994). Thus, there is indication that cultural norms lead Asian Americans to accept as normal a more significant degree of impairment than most, with the result that dementia diagnosis is delayed for a family member until its symptoms become unmanageable. A further illustration is that South Asian culture has no name for dementia (Iliffe & Manthorpe, 2004). Certain cultural models of expected old-age behaviour may include symptoms of dementia as normal aging (Henderson & Henderson, 2002; Teng, 2002). Furthermore, it is frequently mentioned in the mental health literature that there is a tendency for Asian-American groups to somaticize distresses of the mind, in part because of the shame and stigma attached to mental illness (Browne, Fong, & Mokuau, 1994; Sue, 1994; Takamura, 1991). Both normalization of Alzheimer's disease as a correlate of aging and its stigmatization as a form of insanity and cause for shame have been found to impede access to health care services among older adult members of several ethnic minority groups (Ayalon & Arean, 2004; Guo, Levy, Hinton, Weitzman, & Levoff, 2000; Hinton, Guo, Hillygus, & Levkoff, 2000). Furthermore, much like our experience in the Memory Clinic (especially in studies of Asian and Pacific Islander Americans), mental health services have been shown to be underutilized in both inpatient and outpatient settings (Matsuoka, 1990; Sue, 1994)—despite the fact that investigators are convinced that the age-specific prevalence of dementia is similar throughout the world (White, 1992).

Barriers in making an early dementia diagnosis have implications at the patient level, because available medications appear to be relatively more effective in the early stages of the disease and thus more helpful for caregivers. For example, a delay in diagnosis of Alzheimer's disease can negatively impact the ability to manage the condition, affects the quality of life of the patient and of the caregivers, and finally leads to increased resource utilization (Small et al., 1997). Even if it is accepted that dementia can be difficult to diagnosis early in the course of the disease, and, in elderly individuals, sometimes goes unrecognized even if cognitive deterioration has progressed to advanced stage (McCormick, Kukull, van Belle, Bowen, Teri, & Larson, 1994), the balance of evidence is that early diagnosis would greatly assist both patient and the community.

A convincing case exists, then, that ethnic minority elderly are likely to receive the diagnosis of Alzheimer's disease at later stages of the disease, following a long and debilitating illness (Gallagher-Thompson et al., 1997, Guo et al., 2000; Hinton et al., 2000). It follows that, in contexts where more elderly are reluctant to seek help, there will be more patients unlikely to access early interventions and benefit from available treatments. From a treatment perspective, the absolute number of cases of severe dementia will logically increase among ethnic minority elders, with greater strains upon the system. In short, cultural issues will limit the effectiveness of medications since they will be administered late in the disease's history.

NORTHERN ALBERTA RESEARCH ON DEMENTIA AND CULTURE

What had a decisive impact on my personal perception of the role that language itself could play on dementia was the University of Alberta research project on end-of-life care and dementia (see chapter 2 of this volume). The main purpose of the study was to examine how culture affects dementia and end-of-life issues. We were concerned with how dementia was recognized, cared for, and treated in five cultural ethnic communities in Northern Alberta (Cree, francophone, Mandarin-speaking Chinese, Cantonese-speaking Chinese, and Arabic-speaking Muslims of Lac La Biche). During the course of our study, various dimensions of language emerged as particularly significant, even though we had not thought to stress language as we shaped our original questions. Indeed, we did not have language issues as part of our initial questionnaire. Rather, the issue emerged as the team analyzed the results with the facilitator and the liaison people from each group. This engagement with the communities showed that language played a much greater role than we had anticipated. I became sensitized to the many dimensions of language in dementia treatment through this research project. What struck me was the way the language factor was a continuing theme in the data. This data resolved into four key language areas: (1) language and culture influence on disease understanding; (2) second-language difficulties based on translation interaction between health care professional and patients; (3) language reversion in dementia cases; and (4) cultural understandings and their implication for the disease and its acceptance. These issues have been framed as questions in what follows. I must add, however, that these queries also arose in an informal way in my own practice in the Memory Clinic, and hence this research enhanced and corroborated them.

HOW DO LANGUAGE AND/OR CULTURE INFLUENCE
THE UNDERSTANDING OF DEMENTIA?

The Meaning of Mind-Related Disease: Barriers to Assessment and Care

Background information on this topic was surveyed prior to our original study. Much work has been done on Alzheimer's disease. However, we found that cross-ethnic research concerning knowledge of Alzheimer's is limited, and those studies that do exist have relied primarily on qualitative methodology. Researchers have found that, even though the biomedical model of Alzheimer's disease is available, ethnic minorities tend to use folk models to explain Alzheimer's symptomatology (Hinton & Levkoff, 1999; Levkoff, Levy & Weitzman, 1999; Dilworth-Anderson & Gibson 2002). It is reported that the stigma of Alzheimer's disease is prevalent among some ethnic minorities and, in some cases, Alzheimer's disease is seen as a punishment from God (Gallagher-Thompson et al., 2002; Hinton et al., 2000). In addition, Ayalon and Arean (2004) found that certain ethnic minority groups do not have sufficient information about Alzheimer's, so that culturally there is little concern about the disease. There are cases where the language does not support the designation of a dementia illness. Such a case also affects educational potentials—Ayalon and Arean (2004) argue that an extensive evaluation of barriers to knowledge of Alzheimer's disease is needed in order to target minority groups and educate them about Alzheimer's and the importance of early intervention.

Another dimension of this question relates to assessment. Studies have pointed out the major cultural difficulties in the assessment tools utilized among ethnic patients (Torti, Gwyther, Reen, Friedman & Schulman, 2004); furthermore, one study demonstrated that the majority of diagnostic tests on cognitive assessments are not valid within various cultural contexts (Iliffe & Manthorpe, 2004). Indeed, some studies warn physicians that the measurements they use for cognitive abilities (e.g., the Mini-Mental State Examination) often overestimate cognitive impairment in many cultural and linguistic groups (Crum, Anthong, Bassett, & Folstein, 1993; Uhlmann & Larson, 1991).

Ethnic-Specific Distinctions Relating to Dementia in the Northern Study

Nuances of these themes emerged in the research among Chinese, Arabic-speaking Muslims, and francophones. In the Chinese case, various dementias had social implications, since families were held responsible for the well-being of elders. We also found stigmatization applied to specific groups: for example, both Chinese elders and Chinese health care professionals knew cases where lack of English language skills had determined a diagnosis of dementia, when, in fact, the individual was quite articulate in Mandarin and not demented at all. Families, however, were reluctant to challenge physicians' diagnoses when doing so might prejudice the treatment for their loved one if he were seriously ill.

Arabic-speaking Muslims in Lac La Biche had all come from a culture rich in folk traditions. Mental difficulties were also stigmatized, since the advantageous marriage of children depended upon a mental illness-free status within the Lebanese village that was their overseas home. Even when the issue of mate selection did not apply, families were reluctant to acknowledge mental difficulties, preferring to keep the information in a confined inner circle. Also of significance was the fact that common words in Arabic, like *majnun* (mad, out of one's mind), carried great cultural freight that could do individuals a great deal of harm in a small community. There was real concern whether ordinary language comprehension was nuanced sufficiently to deal with dementia. Francophones, in contrast, had no problem with the designation of dementia, but noted that language often played a role in care. Caregiver family members might have little French capability so they could not be relied upon to communicate effectively with an older generation. Moreover, even within a French-speaking community there are regional dialects among older persons, so it may be that caregivers cannot rely on professional interpreters knowing the meaning of some terms. It is obvious that attendance at a memory clinic with English-speaking staff might be ineffective for these ethnic groups.

Indigenous People and Dementia

In the North American Indigenous population, a disease that is "dementing" is relatively new. One reason for this is that this population is only now approaching the life expectancy of the majority population and, consequently, beginning to demonstrate a rising incidence of dementia. In order for the Indigenous population to make sense of the new phenomenon of long-term progressive dementia, it may have to turn to culturally determined explanations to aid in either accepting or coping with such an illness. In fact, beliefs about disease etiology and treatment are important determinants in how persons view the disease and how they respond to advice from health care providers. The more traditional people are, or the less acculturated in their world view and lifestyle, the more likely they are to seek an explanation for their illness within their own cultural frame of reference (Holmes, 1995). Each individual's talk about dementia, for example, reflects biomedical input and cultural understandings framed within the context of the person's unique circumstances and understandings of their experience (Mattingly & Garro, 2000). One Native patient had developed hallucination related to her dementia, along with memory loss, confusion, and impaired ability to recognize her surroundings accurately. The family interpreted the hallucinatory symptoms of dementia as communications with the "other side"; the family did not see her condition as completely pathological. That the hallucinatory symptoms were seen as "supernormal" indicates the positive valence associated with the patient's experience on the "other side." The dementia symptoms of forgetfulness and confused thinking and behaviour are seen as normal outcomes associated with age (Henderson & Henderson, 2002).

We found some of these perceptions to be prevalent among the Cree community who participated in our study. There were around 2,500 Woodland Cree-speaking elders on the Bigstone Reserve, of whom only 50% spoke English. We learned that there was no direct Cree word to designate the illness we identify as dementia, the closest being *wongigiskit*, meaning forgetfulness. Indeed, all the ancillary notions of forgetfulness and memory loss were related to a stage in life, rather than to a disease. The community suggested that to treat such a person as being "ill" was a degradation of their personal worth in their community and removed them from tasks that they could and should be doing.

Moreover, ceremonies are often the purview of the aged in Cree culture, so it was incumbent upon the community to protect these "resource persons" as long as possible. Absent-mindedness at a certain level was regarded as "normal" for those dealing with issues "from the other side." This was the explanation for so little concern about mental competence among seniors. Here was one reason for why elders seldom sought out the Memory Clinic. We also found negative reactions concerning language usage. Elders indicated that they often took medicines and didn't know what they were for, just because they could not understand the medical jargon or comprehend the rationale for taking the drugs provided in English by the physician. In short, we found that cultural and linguistic factors among the Bigstone Cree removed dementia from the list of diseases and made it much more a stage of life related to the elder population, with significant implications for family and community. In this way, language was determining illness and public consciousness of the condition.

HOW SECOND-LANGUAGE ISSUES AND
INTERPRETATION INFLUENCE COMMUNICATION
The Nuance of Language
In the Memory Clinic, the operative language is English. It can now be gathered that some ethnic groups did not access it because their linguistic ability was challenged. However, it is more complicated than that. In our study, we encountered a wide range of issues surrounding second-language use and translation. These were conveyed through discussion with the facilitators of the consensus groups. For example, we learned that there are advantages and disadvantages with different types of interpreters (i.e. family, trained medical, or random). Difficulties in translation may occur at three levels: complex interaction between the interviewer, interpreter, and patient; the mode of receiving the message (direct person-to-person or telephone); and the nature of the mental illness. In my experience, many health care interviewers have doubts about an interpreter's understanding of the questions asked and even more of the answers given, even to the point of wondering whether crucial questions have been asked. The facilitators told us that there are cultural reasons why some kinds of questions will not be asked, or will only be asked in the presence of certain people. Furthermore, there are doubts about the accuracy of the patients' understanding of the questions posed through a translator. Some of the translations may have been coloured by the interpreter's own cultural orientation, or even by his or her experience. Absence of matching vocabulary in some languages posed difficulties, as is obvious in the Cree case. Moreover, facilitators noted that some interpreters requested rephrasing of the question while others improvised; neither process made one very comfortable about the exchange. Clearly, we have no way of gauging how accurate these improvisations are. It became quite logical that someone unsure of his or her English would be reluctant to seek out a Memory Clinic.

Language and Power
Then there were issues of power and authority in translation. Some patients were reluctant to ask questions and clarify issues in the presence of interpreters, because they were known in the community and did not want

personal issues to "go outside." From the point of view of physicians, and certainly in my experience, it was often necessary, but difficult, to observe both the patient and interpreter throughout the interview for non-verbal cues. These cues are important because they indicate whether another agenda is operating beyond the purely medical. Moreover, in a triangular interview, it is sometimes difficult to develop satisfactory rapport that would allow one to evaluate non-verbal cues. Similarly, patients are unable to acknowledge non-verbal cues from the interviewer, a feature found in another study (Shah, 1997).

We experienced other issues when using relatives as translators: patients were reluctant to reveal personal information through their relatives for a variety of reasons, including the risk of the relative having "inside" information and using it "over" the patient. Within the translation situation, the interpretation by relatives had the potential to be biased because the translator sometimes did not him- or herself understand the interviewer's question or the patient's answer, or had poor knowledge of technical terms, had misguided but good intentions, or was culturally antagonistic to the physician's queries (i.e., the interpreter wanted to "protect" the patient from culturally embarrassing questions). Often, the presence of relatives during interviews resulted in a prompting of patients or interference with answers, and posed difficulties in controlling the context of the interview (Shah, 1997). From the best motives, the family may try to protect the patient from bad news, or may decide to tell the patient later in private. Information about side effects may be withheld in the belief that it will improve compliance. As many facilitators from all language groups in our study indicated, family translators often chose not to disclose the extent of a diagnosis to a patient when cultural values discouraged full disclosure of the severity of the disease (Kaufert, 1999).

Occasionally, more sinister reasons may be altering what is said. An abused spouse may want to hide the true cause of his or her injuries. A patient may be inhibited from discussing embarrassing issues or disclosing past events in front of relatives. Despite all these potential issues, I have found that using a relative to translate can have a calming and reassuring influence; also, they are usually readily available, and the patient and interpreter form a cohesive unit against the health care professional. This can be valuable sometimes in assuring that both patient and caregiver have a common perception of the problem.

In many health situations in Alberta, untrained volunteers are often asked to act as interpreters in hospitals; many are the stories of someone being called from the kitchen to help with a language that no one knows. Usually, such interpreters will not have received any training, and though some may have instinctive understanding of what is required, others may be inept, either through lack of empathy or because of a poor grasp of the language. Patients may worry about confidentiality when using an interpreter who is not known to them, especially if they are both members of a small cultural community. Trained interpreters are professionals who maintain a strict code of confidentiality and are skilled in interpreting the sense and intent of what is said while preserving the content of the interview. Their availability and use is still patchy, however, and doctors will often find themselves depending on informal help from friends or relatives of the patient or from untrained volunteers. The bilingual health worker removes the need for a third party to be involved and is the ideal option for most patients (Phelan, 1995). Still, they add a dimension to the health care equation that is not there when health care professional and patient speak the same language, and they are often regarded with hesitancy because they are "on the doctor's side." All of these issues indicate that language translation remains a crucial problem in providing good treatment to patients and proper care to an ethnically diverse population. The difficulties of translation cited in this study allowed me to see why communities with marginal skills in English would be reluctant to seek out staff in a Memory Clinic. At a minimum, they would have little confidence that their case would ever be addressed as they have experienced it. In the worst case, they might feel very vulnerable.

WHAT IMPACT DOES LANGUAGE REVERSION HAVE IN DEMENTIA CASES?

Dementia patients who lose the ability to communicate in their acquired language find communication with their caregivers difficult (Iliffe & Manthorpe, 2004). In a celebrated Edmonton case, a distinguished Albertan suffered from Alzheimer's disease; he was also my patient. He had been raised in China by missionary parents, and his first language was Mandarin. As he progressed into the end-stages of his disease, he reverted back to his first language, that is, to Mandarin. He was able to recite Mandarin poems and was quite articulate in that language. Unfortunately, he was unable to communicate with his family in English, and none knew his first language. Thus, physicians must deal with cases where children of immigrant Alzheimer's patients are not fluent in the homeland's language, while that is the only language their aging parents are able to comprehend. Language reversion means that the end of life can be a very traumatic time for both children and parents.

Similar cases were cited by the facilitator from Peace River dealing with Franco-Albertans. The community members indicated that French dialects were sometimes very difficult to understand because everyone was speaking a contemporary French; few were familiar with a distant dialect of an elderly community member. When a lady who had emigrated from Belgium many years previously was in the end-stage of Alzheimer's in the district, she reverted to an old Belgian-French dialect of her childhood and could not communicate in the French spoken in Alberta. She had been able to speak English at one time, but that language too was lost with the disease. Her daughters were quite unable to communicate with her when she reverted to her original language, much to the dismay of everyone.

Another illustration from my experience is a case drawn from the Chinese community: one Alzheimer's patient spoke a different Chinese dialect from her husband. The children were raised to speak English. When the mother's Alzheimer's disease progressed and the husband died, the children were unable to communicate with her at all. Thus, end-stage care becomes increasingly difficult when language reversion takes place, and caregivers may be unable to convey important information. It is an issue that has to be conveyed to caregivers early in the disease's progress.

Facilitators also noted the problem of accurately communicating informed consent and related information due to language differences. I have found that the inability of patients to appreciate nuances of language sometimes requires caregiver-translators to switch to the worst possible scenario to be sure they are understood, just because of the threat of legal action or some financial encumbrance such as an insurance claim. These exigencies distort the medical case considerably.

CULTURAL UNDERSTANDINGS AND LANGUAGE ISSUES

In effect, then, language features a much larger role in cultural matters of health than I had anticipated in setting up my memory clinic or than we had anticipated when we began our study on the five ethnic communities. For example, several concerns surfaced in our consultations with the Chinese communities. Both Mandarin- and Cantonese-speaking members of the community were concerned that language was a barrier in obtaining services for their seniors and families. For them, language barriers often led to increased inconvenience and anxiety in accessing health care services. They looked to our study to assist them in overcoming some of these. They were hoping for further collaboration with government agencies and other organizations for better use of the existing resources and to train bilingual workers.

The community felt public education was important in accessing this knowledge and resources for aged health care and end-of-life cases. The Chinese community also felt it was important for physicians to respect cultural differences, especially to understand the family pressures to provide as much care as possible for end-of-life patients. The community emphasized the importance of end-of-life situations for maintaining community solidarity and affirming community values. They also suggested that physicians demonstrate some nuance in getting the family to make stressful decisions, since such decisions inevitably had family consequences. It was important to show compassion, respect, and value to an elder, not just to see him or her as an end-of-life case.

Within the francophone population, elders preferred to stay in their community and wanted resources and services consistent with their culture and language. The facilitators noted that there were major differences in attitude depending upon language ability, with second-generation retirees less convinced of their abilities to maintain French culture than the older seniors. This cultural sense had repercussions—it ranged from attitudes about elders aging in place in their communities in order to keep their language and cultural values intact, to concerns whether the next generation would maintain French in a largely English-speaking environment. Alberta francophones had been part of Anglo culture for so long that most of them were thoroughly bilingual and had invested considerably in maintaining their French language and culture.

For all groups, it became increasingly clear that essential health care information should be provided in other languages. Especially when there were issues related to dementia, the gap between what was known and understood by the population, and what was practised in the biomedical community was quite wide. It was also evident that more work will have to be done to provide multilingual environments in Alberta. Otherwise, well-meaning services like the Memory Clinic will continue to miss many people who could benefit from their provisions. With regard to our study, the language dimension of culture is evidently of greater significance in providing health care in Alberta than many had thought, including our team. Perhaps this is a key factor that others researchers may want to build upon.

REFERENCES

American Psychiatric Association. (1994). *Diagnostic and statistical manual of mental disorders* (4th ed.). Washington, D.C.: American Psychiatric Association.

Ayalon, L., & Arean, P.A. (2004). Knowledge of Alzheimer's disease in four ethnic groups of older adults. *International Journal of Geriatric Psychiatry, 19(1)*, 51–57.

Bhatnagar, K.S., & Frank, J. (1997). Psychiatric disorders in elderly from the Indian subcontinent living in Bradford. *International Journal of Geriatric Psychiatry, 12*, 907–12.

Browne, C., Fong, R., & Mokuau, N. (1994). The mental health of Asian and Pacific Islander elders: Implications for mental health administrators. *Journal of Mental Health Administration, 21(1)*, 52–59.

Chrisman, N.J., & Kleinman, A. (1983). Popular health care, social networks, and cultural meanings: The orientation of medical anthropology. In D. Mechanic (Ed.), *Handbook of health, health care, and the health professions* (pp. 569–90). New York: Free Press.

Crum, R.M., Anthong, J.C., Bassett, S.S., & Folstein, M.F. (1993). Population-based norms for the Mini-Mental State Examination by age and educational level. *Journal of the American Medical Association, 269*, 2386–91.

Dilworth-Anderson, P., & Anderson, N.B. (1994). Dementia care giving in blacks: A contextual approach to research. In E. Light, N. Niederhe, B. Lobowitz (Eds.), *Stress effects on family of Alzheimer's patients* (pp. 385–409). New York: Springer.

Dilworth-Anderson, P., & Gibson, B.E. (2002). The cultural influence of values, norms, meanings, and perceptions in understanding dementia in ethnic minorities. *Alzheimer Disease & Associated Disorders, 16(2 Suppl.)*, S56–S63.

Ernst, R.L., & Hay, J.W. (1994). The U.S. economic and social costs of Alzheimer's disease revisited. *American Journal of Public Health, 84*, 1261–64.

Gallagher-Thompson, D., Arean, P.A., Coon, D., et al. (2000). Development and implementation of intervention strategies for culturally diverse care giving populations. In R. Schultz (Ed.), *Handbook on dementia caregiving: Evidence-based interventions for family caregivers* (pp. 151–87). New York : Spring Publishing.

Guo, A., Levy, B.R., Hinton, W.L., Weitzman, P.F., & Levoff, S.E. (2000). The power of labels; Recruiting dementia-affected Chinese American elders and their care-givers. *Journal of Mental Health and Aging, 6*, 103–12.

Henderson, J.M., & Henderson, L.C. (2002). Cultural construction of disease: A "Supernormal" construct of dementia in an American Indian tribe. *Journal of Cross-Cultural Gerontology, 17(3)*, 197–212.

Hinton, W.L., Guo, Z., Hillygus, J., & Levkoff, S. (2000). Working with culture: A qualitative analysis of barriers to recruitment of Chinese-American family caregivers for dementia research. *Journal of Cross-Cultural Gerontology, 15(2)*, 119–37.

Hinton, W.L., & Levkoff, S. (1999). Constructing Alzheimer's: Narratives of lost identities, confusion and loneliness in old age. *Culture, Medicine and Psychiatry, 23(4)*, 453–75.

Hofman, A., Rocca, W.A., Brayne, C., Breteler, M.M., Clarke, M., Cooper, B., et al. (1991). The prevalence of dementia in Europe: A collaborative study of 1980–1990 findings. Eurodem Prevalence European Research Group. *International Journal of Epidemiology, 20(3)*, 736–48.

Holmes, E.R., & Holmes, L.D. (1995). *Other cultures, elder years*. Thousand Oaks, CA; Sage.

Iliffe, S., & Manthorpe, J. (2004). The debate on ethnicity and dementia: From category fallacy to person-centered care? *Aging & Mental Health, 8(4)*, 283–92.

Jones, R.S., Chow, T.W., & Gatz, M. (2006). Asian Americans and Alzheimer's disease: Assimilation, culture and belief. *Journal of Aging Studies, 20*, 11–25.

Kaufert, J.M. (1999). End-of-life decision making among aboriginal Canadians: Interpretation, mediation, and discord in the communication of "bad news." *Journal of Palliative Care, 15(1)*, 31–38.

Levkoff, S., Levy, B., & Weitzman, P.F. (1999). The role of religion and ethnicity in the help seeking of family caregivers of elders with Alzheimer's disease and related disorders. *Journal of Cross-Cultural Gerontology, 14(4)*: 335–56.

Lindesay, J., Jagger, C., Hibbett, M.J., Peet, S.M., & Moledina, F. (1997). Knowledge, uptake and availability of health and social services among Asian Gujarati and white elders. *Ethnicity & Health, 2(1–2)*, 56–69.

Livingston, G., Leavey, G., Kitchen, G., Manela, M., Sembhi, S., & Katona, C. (2001). Mental health of migrant elders—The Islington study. *British Journal of Psychiatry 179*, 361–66.

Mahoney, D.F., Clouterbuck, J., Neary, S., & Zhan, L. (2005). African American, Chinese, and Latino family caregivers' impressions of the onset and diagnosis of dementia: Cross-cultural similarities and differences. *Gerontologist, 45(6)*, 783–92.

Matsuoka, J.K. (1990). Differential acculturation among Vietnamese refugees: Implications for social work practice. *Social Work, 35*, 341–45.

Mattingly, C., & Garro, L.C. (Eds.). (2000). *Narrative and the cultural construction of illness and healing*. Berkeley: University of California Press.

McCormick, W.C., Kukull, W.A., van Belle, G., Bowen, J.D., Teri, L., & Larson, E.B. (1994). Symptom patterns and comorbidity in the early stages of Alzheimer's disease. *Journal of the American Geriatric Society, 42*, 517–21.

McCracken, C.F., Boneham, M.A., Copeland, J.R., Willaims, K.E., Wilson, K., Scott, A., McKibben, P., & Cleave, N. (1997). Prevalence of dementia and depression among elderly people in black and ethnic groups. *British Journal of Psychiatry 171*, 269–73.

Phelan M. (1995). How to do it: Work with an interpreter. *British Medical Journal,*
   311, 555–57.

Shah, A.K. (1997). Interviewing mentally ill ethnic elderly with interpreters.
   Australasian Journal on Ageing, 16(4), 220–21.

Small, G.W., Rabins, P.V., Barry, P.P., Buckholtz, N.S., DeKosky, S.T., Ferris, S.H., et al.
   (1997). Diagnosis and treatment of Alzheimer Disease and related disorders.
   Consensus statement of the American Association of Geriatric Psychiatry,
   the Alzheimer's Association, and the American Geriatrics Society. *Journal*
   of the American Medical Association, 278(16), 1363–71.

Sue, S. (1994). Mental health. In N.W.S. Zane, D.T. Iaeuchi, & K.N.J. Young (Eds.),
   Confronting critical health issues of Asian and Pacific Islander Americans
   (pp. 266–88). Thousand Oaks, CA: Sage.

Takamura, J.C. (1991). Asian and Pacific Islander elderly. In N. Makuau (Ed.),
   Handbook of Social Services for Asian and Pacific Islanders (pp. 185–202).
   New York: Greenwood.

Teng, E.L. (2002). Cultural and educational factors in the diagnosis of dementia.
   Alzheimer Disease and Associated Disorders, 16(2), S77–S79.

Torti, F.M., Gwyther, L.P., Reed, S.D., Friedman, J.Y., & Schulman, K.A. (2004). A multi-
   national review of recent trends and reports in dementia caregiver burden.
   Alzheimer Disease and Associated Disorders, 182, 99–109.

Uhlman, R.F., Larson, E.B. (1991). Effect of education on the Mini-Mental State
   Examination as a screening test for dementia. *Journal of the American Geriatric*
   Society, 39(9), 876–80.

White, L. (1992). Toward a program of cross-cultural research on the epidemiology
   of Alzheimer's disease. *Current Science, 63,* 456–69.

TEN

CULTURAL COMPETENCE OF HEALTH PROFESSIONALS

Olga Szafran MHSA

Earle H. Waugh PhD

Jean A.C. Triscott MD, CCFP, FCFP

INTRODUCTION

Cultural competence has been defined as "a set of congruent behaviours, attitudes, and policies that come together in a system, agency, or among professionals and enables that system, agency, or those professionals to work effectively in cross-cultural situation" (Cross, Bazron, Dennis, & Isaacs, 1989). The goals of culturally competent care include "creat[ing] a health care system and workforce that are capable of delivering the highest-quality care to every patient regardless of race, ethnicity, culture, or language proficiency" (Betancourt, Green, Carrillo, & Park, 2005). Health care professionals trained under the biomedical model and performing under the jurisdiction of various specialized professional associations are understandably challenged by the issue of cultural competence. In the past, ethnic distinctions may have been dealt with as part of the "art" of medicine. Until recently, Western medical training has tried to stay clear of the sets of values and perceptions that patients bring with them (generally under the rubric of "culture" or "ethnicity").

Health professionals are faced with the challenge of caring for patients from many cultures, with different languages, varying socio-economic status, and different understanding of illness and health. All of these issues can affect the amount and kind of care patients receive. In particular, cultural and linguistic barriers are associated with underutilization of health services by patients from ethnically diverse communities (Daker-White, Beattie, Gilliard, & Means, 2002). Moreover, race and ethnicity are factors in patients' perceptions of the medical care they receive (Johnson, Saha, Arbelaez, Beach, & Cooper, 2004) and perceived discrimination is associated with underutilization of health services by patients (Burgess, Ding, Hargreaves, van Ryn, & Phelan, 2008).

Despite the best of intentions, ethnic disparities in health and health services utilization seem to be self-evident. Culturally diverse populations with limited language proficiency have different understandings of health and expectations for care, and different care-seeking behaviours. These perceptions do not necessarily fit well with the way mainstream health care is organized and delivered. In addition, there are health disparities among ethnic minorities. To address health disparities and reduce inequalities, services need to be delivered in a culturally appropriate manner in order to promote service utilization and treatment compliance.

The cultural orientation of health care providers can also influence communication, access, and use of health services. Studies show that bias and stereotyping exists among health professionals (van Ryn & Burke, 2000) and that these traits affect providers' recommendation for use of health services (Schulman et al., 1999; van Ryn, Burgess, Malat, & Griffin, 2006). Furthermore, little research is available on how health professionals perceive and experience their work with patients from ethnically diverse communities. A qualitative study (Kai et al., 2007) in the United Kingdom found that health professionals experienced considerable uncertainty and apprehension when dealing with patients from ethnically diverse backgrounds and were anxious to not appear discriminatory or racist.

A survey of family medicine residency programs in the U.S. revealed that only 28% had a formal multicultural curriculum in place; the remaining 72% had either an informal curriculum or none at all (Culhame-Pera, Like, Lebensohn-Chialvo, & Loewe, 2000). Altshuler, Sussman, and Kachur

(2003) assessed the impact of cultural competence training on intercultural sensitivity in a group of pediatric residents and found that females demonstrated more intercultural sensitivity and benefitted more from intercultural training than male practitioners.

As a modest contribution beyond the paucity of studies on cultural competence in Canadian health professionals, we examined the clinical cultural competence of health professionals working in selected cultural/ethnic communities in northern Alberta within which we had earlier conducted studies in ethnicity and end-of-life and dementia care.

METHODS

Study Design

A self-administered questionnaire survey was used to assess clinical cultural competence of health professionals. This study was phase II of a larger project examining the impact of cultural perspectives on dementia and end-of-life-issues in five communities in Northern Alberta (see chapter 2 in this volume).

Participants and Study Procedures

The sampling frame included 60 health professionals (physicians, nurses, social workers) who provided care to four ethnic/cultural communities in northern Alberta. These communities included the Bigstone Cree in Wabasca, the francophone community in Peace Country Health (McLennan), Lebanese Muslims in Lac La Biche, and Mandarin- and Cantonese-speaking Chinese in Edmonton. While the Cantonese-speaking and Mandarin-speaking Chinese communities considered themselves to be two separate and distinctive cultural groups, the health professionals providing services to the Chinese groups were considered one group. The participants were identified by facilitators in the respective communities. A letter of invitation to attend a culturally responsive care workshop held in the community was mailed to the health professionals, along with the questionnaire and a covering letter describing the survey. Participation was voluntary and consent to take part in the study was implied by the return of a completed questionnaire by mail or fax, or at the workshop. The survey was conducted during May and June 2006. Ethics approval was obtained from the Health Research Ethics Board (Health Panel) of the University of Alberta.

Questionnaire and Data Analysis

The *Clinical Cultural Competence Questionnaire* was employed to assess cultural competence (Like, 2001). The questionnaire was modified for Canadian purposes from self-assessment models developed in the U.S. (Purnell 2002; Goode, Jones, & Mason, 2002; Mason, 1996) and further adapted for Albertan content. It addressed (1) socio-cultural knowledge, (2) skill in dealing with socio-cultural issues, (3) comfort with cross-cultural patient encounters, (4) attitude (awareness, importance), and (5) training in cultural diversity. The questionnaire utilizes a five-point rating scale (1 = not at all, 2 = a little, 3 = somewhat, 4 = quite a bit, 5 = very much) to assess the various elements of cultural competence. Descriptive analysis consisted primarily of frequency distribution and percentages.

RESULTS

A total of 41 completed questionnaires were returned, yielding an overall response rate of 68.3%. The respondents were predominantly female, mean age of 46 years, 58.5% of non-European and 36.6% of European background, predominantly Christian, with 75.6% speaking a second language other than English (table 1).

Socio-cultural Knowledge

The majority (53.8% to 85.4%) of health professionals felt somewhat to not at all knowledgeable about most of the questionnaire items on cultural knowledge (table 2). For 12 out of the 15 items, the most frequent response was "somewhat" knowledgeable, reflecting only a moderate degree of mastery of socio-cultural issues in patient care. Many health care providers were lacking in knowledge with respect to dealing with cross-cultural conflict, compliance, and misunderstandings. Most health professionals also lacked knowledge in assessing health literacy and working with interpreters, as well as knowledge of different healing traditions and ethnopharmacology. Only in the area of socio-cultural issues in geriatrics did the majority (56.1%) of health professionals feel quite a bit to very knowledgeable.

The majority of health professionals felt quite a bit to very skilled at greeting patients in a culturally sensitive manner and providing culturally sensitive end-of-life care (56.1% and 51.3%, respectively) (table 3). Most professionals felt not at all to somewhat skilled at the remaining questionnaire items relating to skill level. Thirty or more per cent felt a little to not at all skilled at eliciting information about the use of folk remedies and alternate healing modalities, the use of folk healers or alternate practitioners, prescribing or negotiating a culturally sensitive treatment plan, and dealing with cross-cultural ethical conflicts.

Comfort with Cross-Cultural Encounters
Over 70% of the health professionals felt quite a bit to very comfortable with caring for patients from culturally diverse backgrounds or those with limited English proficiency, and working with colleagues from culturally diverse backgrounds (table 4). They were least comfortable with patients who make derogatory comments about the health professional's racial or ethnic background, or with colleagues who make derogatory remarks about patients from a particular ethnic group.

Attitude Toward Cross-Cultural Issues in Patient Care
Overwhelmingly, health professionals recognized the importance of socio-cultural issues in interactions with patients, other health professionals, learners, and staff (table 5). Similarly, they indicated that they were quite a bit to very aware of their own racial/ethnic/cultural identity, stereotypes, biases, and prejudices.

Training in Cultural Multicultural Health
While the vast majority (85.4%) of health professionals reported that it was quite a bit to very important for health professionals to receive cross-cultural training, most had received little or no formal cross-cultural training (table 5).

DISCUSSION
The study findings reveal that health professionals recognize the importance that socio-cultural issues have in interactions with patients, colleagues, and learners and are aware of their own cultural identity and biases. Unfortunately, they lack both knowledge of socio-cultural issues and skills in dealing with culturally diverse patient populations. Despite the ethnic diversity in Alberta and the increasing influx of immigrants since the 1950s, it is evident that health professionals have not attained a level of knowledge and skill to effectively relate to patients from culturally diverse backgrounds. Health professionals appear to lack knowledge of different healing traditions and ethnopharmacology, and skill in dealing with the use of folk remedies and healers. This knowledge is necessary

in negotiating a culturally sensitive treatment plan that patients can comply with readily. Particularly problematic is the lack of knowledge in dealing with cross-cultural conflicts, as such conflicts can be time-consuming and anxiety-provoking, and can introduce an element of risk into patient care. It is, however, reassuring that health professionals appear to be skilled at greeting patients in a culturally sensitive manner, as the first few minutes of the doctor–patient encounter can provide the foundation for effective patient-centred care. It is also reassuring that health professionals generally felt skilled at providing culturally sensitive end-of-life care, as the end of life requires an insightful and compassionate understanding of patients' needs and desires.

The health professionals in our study appeared to be quite comfortable with caring for patients who came from culturally diverse backgrounds or had limited English proficiency, and with working with colleagues from culturally diverse backgrounds. These results are as would be expected, implying that Alberta's multicultural social fabric is working. The findings that health professionals are not comfortable with racial or ethnic derogatory marks made by patients or colleagues signify the need for training in dealing with such situations. Health professionals may find it difficult to confront colleagues who make derogatory remarks about patients from a particular ethnic group due to the power structure within the health professionals work environment—that is, they may feel intimidated by their colleagues. There is a need to address this issue in cultural training.

Particularly noteworthy is the finding of a positive attitude toward cultural issues by health professionals in recognizing the importance that culture plays in interactions with patients, colleagues, and learners, and the awareness of their own cultural identity. Perhaps this is a uniquely Canadian finding, reflecting Canada's fundamental principles of multiculturalism and respect for diversity.

Our study findings, which indicate the need for culturally sensitive training within the educational curriculum of health professionals' training, support those of Shaya and Gbarayor (2006). The findings provide direction as to the curriculum content of cultural training for health professionals. This training should include information on different healing traditions, folk remedies, and folk healers; on ethnopharmacology; on how to negotiate a culturally sensitive treatment plan; on dealing with cross-cultural conflict and misunderstanding; on how to assess health literacy and work with interpreters; on socio-cultural issues in mental health and psychiatry; on how the cultural identity of the provider interacts with the cultural identity of the patient; and on approaches to dealing with patients and colleagues who make racially or ethnically derogatory remarks. Kai et al. (2007) also stress that the content-based information in cultural training needs to be addressed and that care must be taken to avoid stereotyping. An awareness of one's own biases is necessary in order to provide culturally sensitive care.

Two Canadian studies have been published on cultural training in health care (Fung, Andermann, Zaretsky, & Lo, 2008; Macdonald, Carnevale, & Razack, 2007), both associating cultural competence with models strongly influenced by an assimilation ideology predominant in the U.S., Australia, and the U.K. While there may be areas of Canadian experience that would find this model helpful, our findings imply that ethnic distinctions are part of the way Canadian culture defines itself. Consequently, cultural features in Canada tend to be much more part of the health care system and are already at play in negotiating diagnosis, treatment, and professional care. At the very least, our study indicates that the Canadian situation requires due awareness of language difficulties in the exchange of health care information.

Cultural training for health professionals should adhere to adult-learning models based on active participation and self-assessment mechanisms. Case-based, interdisciplinary training seemed to be most attractive in the workshops we held and among the groups we worked with. Case-based discussions often led to more nuanced perceptions of the issues, and sometimes indicated where there might be disagreement among participants. The workshop content included the findings from our studies among the ethnic group in their communities. This strategy appears to have won the support of the health care professionals. We suggest that respective cultural communities should have an active role in the development and delivery of the cultural training to health professionals.

Our study has several limitations. The data reflect self-reported perceptions/opinions and the reliability of the responses is unknown. Self-assessments may be subject to distortions and personal biases (Gozu et al., 2007). It is also possible that the respondents may not be representative of others in their profession—that is, they appear to reflect the views of those who are already sensitized to cultural issues. Furthermore, the small sample size and mixed group of health professionals make it difficult to generalize the findings beyond the study sample. In fact, the respondents were from varied Asian, European, and other cultural groups, and were fluent in a variety of languages, thus exhibiting cultural diversity. Thus, while it is not possible to determine the degree of cultural sensitivity bias, its existence would be expected to result in higher scores on knowledge and skills compared to Canadian health professionals overall. An overestimation of the level of cultural competence has been observed by Altshuler, Sussamn, and Kachur (2003). Given that only one specific community was included from each cultural group, the generalizability of the findings beyond the selected communities is unknown.

Studies of the cultural competence of health professionals should employ robust study designs with large sample sizes. The investigation of the cultural competence of a distinct group of health professional at a time, rather than a mixed group, would provide more detailed information of each group and facilitate more targeted training. The content of cultural training should be carefully designed so as to avoid stereotyping of cultural groups, and community input into cultural content is essential. Based on this study, robust evaluations of cultural competence training must be undertaken, including randomized trials of interventions and the development of outcome measures.

AUTHORS' NOTE

This study was funded by the Pallium Project (Phase II) under the aegis of the Primary Health Care Transition Fund, Health Canada. We thank Bunny Bourgeois for assistance on the project.

REFERENCES

Altshuler, L., Sussamn, N.M., & Kachur, E. (2003). Assessing changes in intercultural sensitivity among physician trainees using the intercultural development inventory. *International Journal of Intercultural Relations, 27(4)*, 387–401.

Betancourt, J.B., Green, A.R., Carrillo, J.E., & Park, E.R. (2005). Cultural competence and health care disparities: Key perspectives and trends. *Health Affairs, 24(2)*, 499–505.

Burgess, D.J., Ding, J., Hargreaves, M., van Ryn, M., & Phelan, S. (2008). The association between perceived discrimination and underutilization of needed medical care and mental health care in a multi-ethnic community sample. *Journal of Health Care for the Poor and Underserved, 19(3)*, 894–911.

Cross, T., Bazron, B., Dennis, K., & Isaacs, M. (1989). *Towards a culturally-competent system of care: A monograph on effective services for minority children who are severely emotionally disturbed.* Washington, D.C.: CASSSP Technical Assistance Centre, Georgetown University Child Development Center.

Culhame-Pera, K., Like, R.C., Lebensohn-Chialvo, P., & Loewe R. (2000). Multicultural curricula in family practice residencies. *Family Medicine, 32(3)*, 167–73.

Daker-White, G., Beattie, A.M., Gilliard, J., & Means, R. (2002). Minority ethnic groups in dementia care: A review of service needs, service provision and models of good practice. *Aging & Mental Health, 6(2)*, 101–08.

Fung, K., Andermann, L., Zaretsky, A., & Lo, H.T. (2008). An integrative approach to cultural competence in the psychiatric curriculum. *Academic Psychiatry, 32(4)*, 272–82.

Goode, T., Jones, W., & Mason, J. (2002). A guide to planning and implementing cultural competence organization self-assessment. Washington, D.C.: National Center for Cultural Competence, Georgetown University Child Development Center.

Gozu, A., Beach, M.C., Price, E.G., Gary, T.L., Robinson, K., Palacio A., et al. (2007). Self-administered instruments to measure cultural competence of health professionals: A systematic review. *Teaching and Learning in Medicine, 19(2)*, 180–90.

Johnson, R.L., Saha, S., Arbelaez, J.J., Beach, M.C., & Cooper, L.A. (2004). Racial and ethnic differences in patient perceptions of a bias and cultural competence in health care. *Journal of General Internal Medicine, 19(2)*, 101–10.

Kai, J., Beavan, J., Faull, C., Dodson, L., Gill, P., & Beighton, A. (2007). Professional uncertainty and disempowerment responding to ethnic diversity in health care: A qualitative study. *PLoS Medicine, 4(11)*, 1766–75.

Like, R.C. (2001). Clinical cultural competence questionnaire. Centre for Healthy Families and Cultural Diversity, Department of Family Medicine, UMDNJ—Robert Wood Johnson Medical School. Accessed July 13, 2010, at http://www.umdnj.edu/fmedweb/chfcd/aetna_foundation.htm

Macdonald, M.E., Carnevale, F.A., & Razack, S. (2007). Understanding what residents want and what residents need: the challenge of cultural training in pediatrics. *Medical Teacher, 29(5)*, 444–51.

Mason, J. (1996). *Cultural competence self-assessment questionnaire*. Portland, OR: JLM & Associates.

Purnell, L. (2002). The Purnell model for cultural competence. *Journal of Transcultural Nursing, 13(3)*, 193–96.

Shaya, F.T., & Gbarayor, C.M. (2006). The case for cultural competence in health professions education. *American Journal of Pharmaceutical Education, 70(6)*, 1–6.

Schulman, K.A., Berlin, J.A., Harless, W., Kerner, J.F., Sistrunk, S., Gersh, B.J., et al. (1999). The effect of race and sex on physicians' recommendations for cardiac catherization. *New England Journal of Medicine, 340(8)*, 618–26.

van Ryn, M., Burgess, D., Malat, J., & Griffin, J. (2006). Physicians' perceptions of patients' social and behavioral characteristics and race disparities in treatment recommendations for men with coronary artery disease. *American Journal of Public Health, 96(2)*, 351–57.

van Ryn, M., & Burke, J. (2000). The effect of patient race and socio-economic status on physicians' perception of patients. *Social Science & Medicine, 50*, 813–28.

TABLE 1: *Characteristics of Respondents*

Characteristics	Number n = 41 (%)
Gender	
Female	34 (82.9)
Male	6 (14.6)
Not recorded	1 (2.4)
Age	
≤29 years	4 (9.8)
30–39 years	8 (19.5)
40–49 years	6 (14.6)
50–59 years	8 (19.5)
60+ years	6 (14.6)
Not recorded	9 (22.0)
Ethnic Background	
European	15 (36.6)
Asian	15 (36.6)
First Nations/Métis	6 (14.6)
African	1 (2.4)
Other	2 (4.9)
Not recorded	2 (4.9)
Religion	
Catholic	20 (48.8)
Other Christian	8 (19.5)
Protestant	7 (17.1)
No Religion / Atheist	2 (4.9)
Other	2 (4.9)
Muslim	1 (2.4)
Not recorded	1 (2.4)
Lived/Visited Outside of Canada	26 (38.7)
Speak a Language Other than English	31 (75.6)
Language Spoken (n = 31)	
Chinese (Mandarin, Cantonese)	12 (38.7)
French	10 (32.3)
Cree	5 (16.1)
Filipino	2 (6.5)
Nigerian	1 (3.2)
Not recorded	1 (3.2)

TABLE 2: *Clinical Cultural Knowledge of Health Professionals*

Health Professionals' Knowledge About...	Knowledge Level n = 41 (%)*		
	Not At All/ A Little	Somewhat	Quite a Bit/Very
1. Demographics of diverse racial/ ethnic groups	22.0	43.9	34.1
2. Socio-cultural characteristics of diverse racial or ethnic groups	19.5	48.8	31.7
3. Health risks experienced by diverse racial or ethnic groups (n = 40)	17.5	42.5	40.0
4. Health disparities experienced by diverse racial or ethnic groups	24.4	34.1	41.5
5. Socio-cultural issues in			
Geriatrics	9.8	34.1	56.1
Psychiatry (n = 37)	32.4	35.1	32.4
Women's Health (n = 37)	18.9	40.5	40.5
6. Ethnopharmacology	53.7	31.7	14.6
7. Different healing traditions (n = 40)	30.0	40.0	30.0
8. Historical and contemporary impact of racism, bias, prejudice, and discrimination in health care experienced by various population groups in Canada	19.5	48.8	31.7
9. Providing culturally sensitive clinical preventative services (n = 39)	25.6	28.2	45.2
10. Providing culturally sensitive end-of-life care (n = 39)	23.1	25.6	51.3
11. Assessing health literacy (n = 39)	20.5	43.6	35.9
12. Working with medical interpreters (n = 39)	20.5	41.0	38.5
13. Dealing with cross-culture conflicts relating to diagnosis/treatment	29.3	39.0	31.7
14. Dealing with cross-cultural adherence/ compliance problems (n = 40)	22.5	47.5	30.0
15. Dealing with cross-cultural ethical conflicts (n = 39)	30.8	43.6	25.6
16. Apologizing for cross-cultural misunderstanding or errors (n = 38)	28.9	36.8	34.2

* *Percentage calculated out of n = 41, except where noted otherwise.*

TABLE 3: *Clinical Cultural Skill of Health Professionals*

Health Professionals' Skill in Dealing with...	Skill Level n = 41 (%)*		
	Not At All/ A Little	Somewhat	Quite a Bit/Very
1. Greeting patients in a culturally sensitive manner	7.3	36.6	56.1
2. Eliciting the patient's perspective about health and illness	17.1	34.1	48.8
3. Eliciting information about the use of folk remedies and/or alternative healing modalities (n = 40)	37.5	25.0	37.5
4. Eliciting information about the use of folk healers and/or alternative practitioners (n = 40)	40.0	30.0	30.0
5. Performing a culturally sensitive physical examination (n = 39)	25.6	38.5	35.9
6. Prescribing or negotiating a culturally sensitive treatment plan (n = 40)	30.0	35.0	35.0
7. Providing culturally sensitive patient education or counselling (n = 39)	23.1	33.3	43.8
8. Providing culturally sensitive clinical preventative services (n = 39)	25.6	28.2	46.2
9. Providing culturally sensitive end-of-life care (n = 39)	23.1	25.6	51.3
10. Assessing health literacy (n = 39)	20.5	43.6	35.9
11. Working with medical interpreters (n = 39)	20.5	41.0	38.5
12. Dealing with cross-cultural conflicts relating to diagnosis or treatment	29.3	39.0	31.7
13. Dealing with cross-cultural adherence compliance problems (n = 40)	22.5	47.5	30.0
14. Dealing with cross-cultural ethical conflicts (n = 39)	30.8	43.6	25.6
15. Apologizing for cross-cultural misunderstanding or errors (n = 38)	28.9	36.8	34.2

* Percentage calculated out of n = 41, except where noted otherwise.

TABLE 4: *Comfort Level of Health Professionals in Dealing with Cross-Cultural Encounters/Situations*

Health Professionals' Comfort with...	Comfort Level n = 41 (%)*		
	Not At All/ A Little	Somewhat	Quite a Bit/ Very
1. Caring for patients from culturally diverse backgrounds	12.2	9.8	78.0
2. Caring for patients with limited English proficiency	7.3	22.0	70.7
3. Caring for a patient who insists on using or seeking folk healers or alternative therapies (n = 40)	12.5	35.0	52.5
4. Identifying beliefs that are not expressed by a patient or caregiver, but might interfere with the treatment regimen (n = 39)	17.9	41.0	41.0
5. Being attentive to non-verbal cues or the use of culturally specific gestures that might have different meanings in different cultures (n = 40)	27.5	30.0	42.5
6. Interpreting different cultural expressions of pain, distress, and suffering	22.0	31.7	46.3
7. Advising a patient to change behaviours or practices related to cultural beliefs that impair one's health (n = 39)	30.8	35.9	33.3
8. Speaking in an indirect rather than a direct way to a patient about his or her illness, if this is more culturally appropriate (n = 39)	28.2	41.0	30.8
9. Breaking "bad news" to a patient's family first, rather than to a patient, if this is more culturally appropriate (n = 36)	27.8	36.1	36.1
10. Working with health professionals from culturally diverse backgrounds (n = 40)	10.0	17.5	72.5
11. Working with a colleague who makes derogatory remarks about patients from a particular ethnic group (n = 39)	48.7	28.2	23.1
12. Treating a patient who makes derogatory comments about your racial/ethnic background	43.6	25.6	30.8

* Percentage calculated out of n = 41, except where noted otherwise.

TABLE 5: *Health Professionals' Attitude Toward and Training in Cultural Issues*

	Level of Importance n = 41 (%)*		
Importance of socio-cultural issues in interaction with...	**Not At All/ A Little**	**Quite a Bit/Very**	**Quite a Bit/Very**
Patients	4.9	14.6	80.5
Health professional colleagues	7.3	29.3	63.4
Residents and medical students (n = 39)	10.3	28.2	61.5
Staff	4.9	29.3	65.9
Awareness of your own...			
Racial, ethnic, or cultural identity (n = 39)	2.6	7.7	89.7
Racial, ethnic, or cultural stereotypes (n = 39)	2.6	10.3	87.2
Biases and prejudices	7.7	15.4	76.9
Importance for health professionals to receive training in cultural diversity or multicultural health care	0.0	14.6	85.4
Amount of training in cultural diversity health professionals previously received in...			
College/post-secondary education (n = 35)	45.7	34.3	20.0
University (n = 29)	55.2	31.0	13.8
Medical school (n = 14)	57.1	28.6	14.3
Residency training (n = 16)	56.3	25.0	18.8
Continuing professional education (n = 36)	30.6	30.6	38.9

* Percentage calculated out of n = 41, except where noted otherwise.

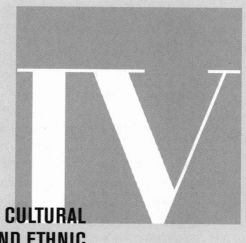

IV

**CULTURAL
AND ETHNIC
DIVERSITY IN
HEALTH CARE**

OVERVIEW

Diversity is a fundamental characteristic of Canadian society. Canada's multicultural society has been shaped over time by over 50 different Aboriginal groups indigenous to the country, followed by waves of immigrants, primarily from Europe, Asia, and Africa, and their descendants. Canada's visible minority population is growing at a faster rate than its total population. Multiculturalism has not only created demographic diversity, but also diversity of values and cultural perspectives. Cultural and ethnic groups differ in how health is viewed, which health services are utilized, and how ill health is managed. This part of the book presents different cultural and ethnic perspectives on health and health practices, using diverse methodological approaches.

In "Cultures of Menopause in an Ethnically Diverse Society: Biomedical Perspectives, Women's Perspectives," Denise Spitzer examines the biomedical and ethno-socio-cultural perspectives of menopause and how they interact. She uses a life history approach to examine the impact of immigration on Chinese-, Somali-, and Chilean-Canadian women's experience of menopause. The meanings of menopause are embedded in cultural, personal, and highly flexible individual perspectives.

In "Health and Health Care Utilization Patterns of Visible Minority Seniors in Canada," Juhee Suwal conducts a quantitative comparison of health and health services utilization of visible minorities versus White seniors in Canada. Differences in perceived health and health services utilization between visible minorities and White seniors are explained in terms of cultural and economic differences between these groups. Given the inability to sub-classify the various cultural and ethnic groups within the visible minority group, "culture" is explored in a broad context in this chapter.

David Young uses participant observation in his work on "Aboriginal Healing." He discusses the methods he employed as an anthropologist in researching Aboriginal healing over a number of years, and the controversy associated with some of these methods in the area of objective science. Based on his work on Aboriginal healing, Young argues that the study of the healing practices of a cultural group requires a great deal of commitment, the process may change the researcher's values and personality, and it may be fraught with suspicion on the part of the cultural group. Despite these challenges, documentation of traditional knowledge and healing practices will enhance our understanding of the holistic nature of health. Young's work also implies that the understanding of various cultural perspectives requires individuals to be open to differing beliefs and practices, and have a tolerance and respect for differences.

In "Reflections of a Cree Healer's Partner," Delores Cardinal reflects on the role of the Aboriginal healer's wife, a topic that has received only scant attention in the literature to date. Her reflection is an important step in beginning to document traditional healing practices among the Cree people. Delores Cardinal points out that such healing is always a fusion of elements: learned lore; respect for plants, animals, and humans; and loyalty to spiritual sources that have granted the original knowledge. A partner in this process, she is "gifted" in the Aboriginal way; the talent brings with it concomitant responsibility. It is evident that, in the healing protocols, husband and wife act as a seamless team, rising above their distinctive personalities to bring relief to their people.

ELEVEN

CULTURES OF MENOPAUSE IN AN ETHNICALLY DIVERSE SOCIETY

BIOMEDICAL PERSPECTIVES, WOMEN'S PERSPECTIVES

Denise L. Spitzer PhD

MENOPAUSE IS A UNIVERSAL FEMALE phenomenon marked by the cessation of menstruation. This biological event and the somatic responses with which it is sometimes associated are imbued with cultural meanings that may be personally or collectively constructed. Focusing on symptoms or a disease model of menopause, however, greatly underestimates women's attribution of meanings to, and experiences of, the change of life; instead, the menopausal transition must be considered in a broader scope of women's lives. Indeed, cultural differences pertaining to menopause emerge as much along the professional–patient divide as they do along more widely acknowledged ethnic divisions. For health professionals hoping to understand the needs of mid-life women from various cultural communities, an appreciation of the dynamic cultural, economic, and personal factors that help shape all women's experience of menopause is essential.

INTRODUCTION

Over 700 million women around the world have transitioned into the post-reproductive phases of their lives known as menopause (Diczfalusy, 1986). The vast numbers of women who have entered this phase of their lives, coupled with higher rates of international immigration and transnational linkages, have contributed to a burgeoning interest in menopause from a cross-cultural perspective. In particular, ethnically diverse and aging populations such as Canada's have served as sites where immigrant and refugee women and physicians potentially confront disparate notions of aging and menopause.

In this chapter, I examine the biomedical and ethno-cultural constructions of menopause and consider how these constructs interact. I begin with an overview of the development of biomedical perspectives on menopause from Aristotle to hormone replacement therapy (HRT). Next I offer a brief tour of the socio-cultural research on menopause and highlight my own research with Chinese-, Somali-, and Chilean-Canadian women and their experiences of menopause and maturation in their new society. I conclude with a discussion of the ways in which these perspectives intersect and challenge each other.

BIOMEDICAL PERSPECTIVES ON MENOPAUSE

While biomedicine is not a homogenous practice, its historical roots inform commonly held perspectives on women's health, women's bodies, and aging. Cessation of menses is mentioned in texts attributed to Aristotle and Pliny the Elder nearly two thousand years ago and in the medieval writings of Hildegard von Bingen (Amundsen and Diers, 1970, 1973); the term *la ménopause*, however, was first noted in a French medical text dating back to 1823 (Wilbush, 1986). European medical texts from the fourteenth through eighteenth centuries regarded menstrual blood as a pure substance vital to nurturing the fetus in utero and cleansing the female body (Bynum, 1991); "if, however, it is retained too long—it offends in Quality" (Aristotle, 1763, p. 29). The retention of menstrual blood was thought to lead to the accumulation of bodily toxins that would corrupt women's bodies. By the closing of the eighteenth century, most French medical texts referred to this stage of women's lives as *le temps critique* or *l'enfer des femmes* (Wilbush, 1986). The notion that menopause was a widespread female malady was refined in subsequent centuries when the medical model of menopause was further entrenched. Edward Tilt, a British physician who studied in France in the

1830s, brought the French notions of menopause into the English-speaking medical world. According to Tilt, there were well over a hundred symptoms associated with the change of life, which represented both a crisis and a return to a normal, masculine state of being (Wilbush, 1980).

All women were not, however, equal. Thomas (1880) wrote that women not exposed to the deprecating influences of civilization could compete with men as their equals, just as in forms of lower animals. Another medical text of the period stated,

> The civilized woman differs both physically and socially from her barbarous sister, and from the female of the lower animals, in many important particulars. She is more liable to the pathological conditions which, more or less, all females have in common. These conditions appear in a more severe form, and are followed by more disastrous results, in the civilized than in the barbarous state. (Penrose, 1900, p. 17)

He goes on to suggest that overwork of the brain and excessive development of the nervous system, improprieties of dress, contraception, and abortion all contribute to women's ill health.

The manner in which young women dealt with the onset of menstruation was believed to have implications for their health status at menopause. In the Victorian era, the body was viewed as a closed energy system, analogous to a machine whose task was to reproduce (Barbe, 1993; Martin, 1987). Any effort that detracted energy from this path would diminish women's capacity to function, or to perform their functions adequately, and could cause them to lose control of their reproductive duties and their lives. For instance, young girls who were subjected to too much mental strain or who expressed sexual desires were in jeopardy of losing the delicate balance between their nerves and muscles, leading to painful menstrual cycles and potentially to insanity, hysteria, tuberculosis, vaginal inflammation, and cancer as they approached the end of their menstrual lives (Barbe, 1993; Penrose, 1900; Smith-Rosenberg, 1985). This relationship between medicine, menopause, gender, and social control was well entrenched with the onset of the development of menopause as a biomedical construct as physicians' advice to women functioned to constrain their personal and social behaviour.

The transition to the twentieth century brought changes to women's status and to biomedical constructions of menopause. While both positive and negative images of menopausal women circulated in popular North American discourse, concerns persisted that post-menopausal women would pathologically pursue youthful attributes or express inappropriate sexual desires (Banner, 1992).

In the 1930s, two major turns in scientific advancement greatly contributed to the discursive shaping of menopause, menopausal women, and the menopausal body from a biomedical perspective. The emergence of endocrinology and gynaecology, aided by the pharmaceutical industry, helped to forge the notion that hormones were in essence the messengers of gender (Oudshoorn, 1994). It followed then that menopause became construed as an endocrine deficiency disease, laying the foundation for the development of hormonal supplements to restore a woman to her "natural" state; by the 1940s, Premarin was marketed for the relief of menopausal symptoms (Rousseau, 2002; Spitzer, 2003). Concomitantly, the field of psychology gained credibility. The foremost female Freudian psychologist of the day, Helene Deutsch, proclaimed that post-menopausal women experienced a partial death as they encountered their post-reproductive years, and like some physicians in previous decades, she decried the behaviour of the pathetic older woman desperate to seduce a younger man (Deutsch, 1945). The loss of reproductive potential could lead to severe depression given the disease label of involutional melancholia. While increasing numbers of mid-life women were diagnosed with this condition, some mental health specialists challenged the veracity of the label. Many of the clients referred to them were still menstruating regularly or lacked the symptoms associated with the syndrome and appeared for the most part to need someone with whom they could speak about their problems (Donovan, 1951; Greenhill, 1946). Despite an evident gap between women's experiences and complaints of menopause, and biomedical knowledge and physician advice, experts continued to warn that an "asymptomatic menopause may initiate silent, progressive and ultimately lethal sequelae" (cited in Barbe, 1993, p. 32).

The panacea to avoid these potentially dangerous outcomes was of course estrogen replacement therapy. As Fausto-Sterling (1999) has noted, biomedicine focused on the potency of estrogen, the quintessential female hormone, because biomedicine is always searching for a singular cause and effect. When in the mid-1970s unopposed estrogen was found to increase risks of endometrial cancer, combined estrogen and progester-one therapies were marketed (Rousseau 2002). Although population-based surveys repeatedly demonstrated that only a minority of women suffer from menopausal complaints sufficiently severe to prompt consultation with a physician and that only vasomotor symptoms are associated with menopausal status (Avis, Brockwell, & Colvin, 2005; Kaufert, 1980), bio-medical advice to mid-life women focused on the use of HRT to not only mitigate symptoms, but also as a prophylaxis against a growing number of illnesses from heart disease to Alzheimer's (Rousseau, 2002; Spitzer, 2003). In 1993, for instance, the American College of Physicians, the American College of Family Medicine, and the U.S. Preventative Services Task Force (USPSTF) issued guidelines that urged health care providers to prescribe HRT for women at risk of heart disease and osteoporosis (Rousseau, 2002). Physicians and pharmaceutical companies decried what they perceived as underuse of HRT, which they held as, on balance, greatly beneficial to women (Jolly, 1997; Odens et al., 1992; Spitzer, 2003).

The promulgation of HRT as the key to women's good health in their mature years stalled considerably with the publication of the results of two major randomized controlled trials: Heart and Estrogen/Progestin Replacement Study (HERS) I and II and the Women's Health Initiative (WHI). The HERS trials included women with coronary heart disease to determine whether HRT would offer protection against future coronary events; however, in the first year the group that received HRT reported 52% more heart disease along with higher levels of venous thromboembolism and gallbladder disease than the control group (Gupta & Aronow, 2002; Humphries & Gill, 2003; Manson & Martin, 2001; North American Meno-pause Society, 2002). The WHI, which enrolled over 161,000 women at 40 clinics, was the first major randomized controlled trial many believed would silence the HRT skeptics once and for all (see WHI, 2002). After an average of five years of follow-up with 16,608 women, the estrogen plus progester-one versus placebo arm of the WHI trial was halted by an independent Data and Safety Monitoring Board due to adverse effects (Kuller, 2003; Lemay, 2002; Piantadosi, 2003; Schneider, 2002). Increased hazard ratios for coro-nary heart disease, stroke, breast cancer, and pulmonary embolism were reported (Kuller, 2003); for example, the risk of stroke increased in year two and persisted through year five of the WHI study (WHI, 2002). Those with estrogen and progestin had higher rates of invasive breast cancer and were diagnosed at more advanced stage (Chelebowski et al., 2003).

The results of these trials have altered women's uptake of HRT and clinical guidelines for its use (Canada NewsWire, 2003; USPSTF, 2003; Society of Obstetricians and Gynaecologists of Canada [SOGC], 2003, 2006). The most recent consensus report from the Society of Obstetricians and Gynaecologists of Canada suggests that "Healthcare providers should offer HT (ET/estrogen-progestin therapy) as the most effective therapy for the medical management of menopausal symptoms" (SOGC, 2006, p. 16). HRT is recommended for the treatment of moderate to severe symptoms and should not be employed for the prevention of cardiovascular disease or dementia. It should be prescribed for an "appropriate duration to achieve treatment goals at the lowest effective dose" (p. 16). Thus, HRT still remains a panacea, although it is approached with greater caution. Menopause is still regarded as a medical concern with symptoms and sequelae that demand intervention (Murtagh & Hepworth, 2003b). Current medical guidelines also include lifestyle counselling recommending that women take up gardening, breathing exercises, reduce stress, and attend to their diets (SOCG, 2006). This focus on self-care not only reinforces individualism and individual responsibility for the body, laying the responsibility of risk prevention on the bodies of women (Murtagh & Hepworth, 2003a), but it also presumes a certain class position where women can afford the time and money to indulge in self-care activities (Anderson, Blue, & Lau, 1991; Spitzer, 1995, 2003).

In summary, biomedical perspectives remain focused on menopause as a condition worthy of medical consideration and intervention in the shape of hormone (replacement) therapy. While the amelioration of symptoms remains at the core of biomedical interests, it is still predicated on a static, universal female menopausal body while the diversity of women, their experiences, and their perspectives are not taken into account (Murtagh & Hepworth, 2003a; Spitzer, 1995).

SOCIO-CULTURAL PERSPECTIVES ON MENOPAUSE

How do women experience menopause? Is it a universal experience or are there cultural and personal variations? We live in the sensate world of our bodies and learn to interpret, label, and grant meaning to somatic stirrings through our interactions with others in the intersubjective space of shared meaning that is culture. Thus, women may not consciously attend to a rise in body temperature and the appearance of sweat at different times of their lives depending on activity levels. The same physiological responses that may be interpreted as hot flashes as women go through peri- and post-menopause may not be consciously labelled or similarly attributed when women are breastfeeding or simply in the luteal phase of their menstrual cycle. Csordas refers to somatic modes of attention that "are culturally elaborated ways of attending to and with one's body in surroundings that include the embodied presence of others" (2002, p. 244).

The constellation of signs and symptoms associated with the cessation of menstruation—and the meaning assigned to this life event—differ cross-culturally and individually. In Japan, *konenki* is period of time that can last from an average of 6.7 years to up to 10 years and is associated with aging; the end of menstruation is just part of the process (Lock, 1993; Rosenberger, 1986). It is considered a "luxury disease" by physicians, who maintain that women active in fulfilling appropriate, gendered caregiving roles are less apt to acquire it; symptoms include sore shoulders, tingling, irritability, and chills (Lock, 1993; Lock, Kaufert, & Gilbert 1988). In China, *geng nian qi* (change of years) is a similar transition; less than half of women surveyed experienced low to moderate symptoms (Shea, 2006). Shiu-Yun et al. (2003) found that over one-third of the Taiwanese women and one-quarter of Australian women they surveyed had no particular feelings about menopause whatsoever. In addition, over 47% of the Australian and 32% of the Taiwanese women expressed explicit relief about the cessation of menses.

The timing of menopause can be of great importance. If women feel that their childbearing is incomplete, menopause may be more troubling; however, for many women and in many cultures—for instance women of the Mohawk Nation—menopause is a time for themselves (Bruce & Gottlieb, 1991). Moreover, the anticipation of menopause may be accompanied by greater fear and negative feelings than going through the transition itself. For instance, Sampselle et al. (2002) found that African-American women generally viewed menopause as a natural part of life and did not assign any negative value to the event, although younger women approached it with greater trepidation. Menopause was not even identified as a major life event. Indeed, physicians and mid-life women may in general possess disparate perspectives of menopause when it is placed in the context of women's lives. When asked to identify the major problems faced by mid-life women, over 20% of physicians listed menopause while none of the mid-life women mentioned it. Furthermore, 60% of the mid-life women and 17% of the physicians agreed that menopause was of no concern to middle-aged women (DeLorey, 1992).

THE MENOPAUSAL EXPERIENCES OF CHINESE-, SOMALI-, AND CHILEAN-CANADIAN WOMEN

I undertook qualitative research, employing a life history approach, to deepen my understanding of women's experiences of menopause and specifically to explore those experiences in the context of immigration. In life history research, the focus is on the participant as an actor in her life and social world. The approach allows retrospective reflection and is well-suited to placing issues in the context of the life cycle (Watson & Watson-Franke, 1985). For this study, 33 women—11 each from Somalia, China, and Chile—were recruited. These three communities were selected as they differed in size and timing of immigration, degree of acculturation to the Canadian environment, and development of ethnic infrastructure. Women were recruited for the study via network sampling. Interviews were held in the language of the woman's choice and took place in Edmonton, Toronto, and Ottawa.

Chinese-Canadian Women

The Chinese-Canadian women in the study regarded menopause as a natural event; it did not give a woman cause for concern, and in fact, women could feel in better health and free from the annoyances of the menstrual cycle. Informants noted that in China, few women consult a physician at menopause. Although most felt that discussion of menopause was restricted in their mother's generation, these women were talking openly with friends, co-workers, and spouses about their experiences. Most assumed that all women's experiences were similar; however, the level of intensity that women encountered might be different.

To apprehend the dominant cultural construct of menopause, I asked informants to describe the attributes they associated with this term. The Chinese participants offered a list of symptoms in descending order of frequency: hot flashes, irregular or heavy bleeding, mood changes or bad temperament, insomnia, irregular heartbeat, vaginal dryness, rashes, sweating, overall bodily pain, decreased libido, and weight gain. In their personal experience, few had more than a handful of symptoms. Several women sought out traditional Chinese herbs such as dong quai to address the imbalances in their system that gave rise to symptom expression. Some of the informants who were themselves physicians reported prescribing dong quai, other herbal preparations, and sleeping pills to patients suffering from insomnia. They noted that HRT was available in China but seldom used.

Importantly, private distress (due to the death of loved ones or the tribulations of immigration) or more public stress (from political condemnation that was a feature of the Great Proletarian Cultural Revolution [1966–1976]) that occurred concomitantly with the menopausal transition resulted in suffering that suffused through the body and somatic symptoms of menopause. Given the absence of mind/body dichotomy in traditional Chinese medical thought, there was no need to disentangle which symptoms were attributable to menopause and which others had origins in more generalized stress response. For instance, Lai Ming[1] had lost one child to diphtheria; when her other children contracted the disease, she succumbed to a host of symptoms that were treated with a variety of tranquilizers and antidepressants:

> I could not distinguish whether it was menopause or I was too
> concerned and nervous about anything. Therefore, when I lost
> my temper, they would say I had menopause. When I experienced
> hot flashes, I went to the doctor. The doctor confirmed that I was
> having menopause.

For many of the Chinese-Canadian women interviewed, menopause also heralded a second youth, a time when the children are grown but without children of their own, a time to be increasingly active in social, spiritual, and personal activities. The women who had more recently immigrated from China, however, emphasized that education and environment influenced how women would experience this time of life. Educated urban women were seen as those most able to enjoy this second youth, devoting themselves to learning calligraphy or drawing, while less educated individuals or those in rural areas would still be compelled to labour or take on greater responsibility in the home.

Recent immigration to Canada had a significant impact on the menopausal years of these women. Rather than contributing to society through work, many were unemployed; rather than enjoying their second youth learning traditional arts or visiting friends, many were physically, linguistically, or economically isolated. This isolation was still evident even when women were living with their families, as intergenerational struggles were fought with little support for their point of view. The women who had been in Canada the longest were more adept at adjusting to menopause in the Canadian context, seeing this period as a time to let their children go, enjoy their spouse and friends, or devote themselves to personal or community activities.

Chilean-Canadian Women

None of the Chilean-Canadian women I interviewed were concerned with the loss of their reproductive potential, although a few felt that other women more interested in having more children might find menopause difficult for that reason. As with menstruation, menopause in Chile had been very secretive although some noted that degrading jokes about menopausal women were common in Chilean society. In contrast to their mothers' generation, the mid-life Chilean-Canadian informants were interested in talking to other women and actively seeking out a cohort of friends to support each other through the transition. Many shared the same perspective as their mothers, who regarded menopause as synonymous with aging.

This group of informants also presented the most elaborate list of complaints that they associated with the menopausal transition. Hot flashes, moodiness, erratic bleeding, headaches, nausea, depression, nervousness, vaginal dryness, lack of concentration, changes in skin elasticity, feelings of heaviness, shortness of breath, generalized tendency to become ill, fragile bones, and weight gain were cited as the symptoms associated with menopause. Again, it is important to note that informants did not report experiencing all of these symptoms; instead, the list reflects the construction of a menopausal syndrome that circulated in the dominant Chilean-Canadian discourse.

Women generally regarded the occurrence of menopausal symptoms as inextricably linked to their lives as women—and more specifically as immigrant women. For example, one woman experienced a variety of complaints that her friends, colleagues, and physician attributed to menopause; when she divorced her husband of 20 years, the symptoms disappeared (Spitzer, 2009). Another noted that the insomnia she suffered, interpreted by her physician as a menopausal symptom, was from her perspective rooted in financial worries that were directly linked to the process of deskilling that she and her husband have undergone while living in Canada for 20 years (Spitzer, 2009).

Living out their lives in Canada was not a part of Chilean-Canadian women's dreams. Circumstances forced most of them to flee their homeland after the 1973 military coup and find refuge in Canada, for which they were most grateful. Torn from family and friends, their expectations of becoming grandmothers caring for grandchildren or retiring at age 55 have not been realized. In Canada, these women were finding new meanings for themselves in their menopausal years by extending their work life and engaging in a period of self-reflection and creativity. Some were reassessing their marriages, others were spending time on artistic endeavours, and many were seeking out the company of other Chilean women to share their experiences. As Christina said,

> I read all these stories about how women get depressed and I was
> aware of all that. I always thought that's not going to happen to me.
> I was prepared for that; I truly did [sic]. I was the one who brought
> in that subject with friends: "we shouldn't do this, we shouldn't
> let this. We're perfect, we're beautiful, we're everything." (Spitzer,
> 2007, p. 56)

Somali-Canadian Women

The Somali term for menopause, *dhaqmo ka bax*, literally means "unlikely to bear children." Childbearing is of paramount importance to Somali culture; therefore, one might assume that the end of reproductive life might be problematic for women. However, the end of menstruation is considered good when a woman is past the age when it is regarded as safe or considered appropriate to bear children. Some women mentioned that other women they heard about refused to believe they were going through menopause, insisting they were pregnant or experiencing a miscarriage. For themselves, however, menopause was consistently regarded as the "best time of your life," a time of independence and no cause for concern. Most importantly, post-menopausal women are fully able to devote themselves to prayer and study of the Qu'ran.

Aisha, a mother of eight children, summed up the attitude of the women I spoke with:

> Thank God, when you have the period you don't feel *daahir*, you
> don't feel comfortable, you don't feel deeply clean to pray. So if

you are not *daahir*...you don't go to the mosque, you can't touch the Qu'ran, the holy Qu'ran book....we accept it and it's just part of life.... [At menopause] your children grow up, so you don't care about husbands and you don't care about having periods. We don't care about any of this...we don't care about the husbands, sleeping with them, or the period!

Few somatic symptoms were associated with the Somali construction of menopause. Only one woman reported experiencing a menopausal symptom—heavy bleeding at the onset of perimenopause; the remainder did not personally recall any symptoms associated with the transition although several had heard that women might experience painful breasts, cramps, or changes in temperament. Furthermore, menopause was not a marker for old age. After age 40, women are considered elders and are addressed by the term *erdo* or Auntie. Women are regarded as old in their sixties or seventies when they take on the role of grandmother and are treated with great esteem.

Post-menopausal Somali women were able to re-create certain areas of their lives in Canada, such as seeking out the companionship of other women of the same age to study and pray; however, the grandmother role was more elusive. For those whose children are not in Canada, the situation is obvious. Others had some or all of their children with them and were confronting new intergenerational tensions: children wanted to date members of the opposite sex or move away from home, or were not eager to marry, thus circumventing their mothers' expectations for their offspring and themselves. Still, they were adapting to new possibilities, as one woman announced in the presence of her daughter, "As soon as all of you finish university, I'm moving to Mecca, forget about taking care of grandchildren!"

CULTURES OF MENOPAUSE

Biomedicine is informed by scientific principles of empiricism and objectivity, and reflects the values of individualism and the uniformity of the body (Freund & McGuire, 1995; Gordon, 1988). My brief overview of biomedical perspectives on menopause suggests that historical, economic, political, and social contexts have significant roles to play in shaping medical advice and interventions, and the dominant discursive constructions of menopause and the menopausal body. Focusing on symptoms and the mitigation thereof, biomedicine has offered HRT as a solution, accompanied by the recent inclusion of recommendations for lifestyle alterations that are predicated on middle-class, Euro-Canadian values of individualism and leisure.

However, as numerous studies of diverse groups of women suggest, menopause is not generally regarded as a critical time in women's life requiring medical intervention. This is not to suggest that some women do not experience troublesome symptoms for which they may seek out self-medication, other self-care solutions, or the assistance of a physician; nor is it to suggest that some women (albeit a minority) might not experience severe symptoms that may be disruptive to their lives. Symptom expression, however, does not reflect the totality of women's perspectives on menopause. In a review of the literature pertaining to menopause in 96 cultures, I found that the presence of symptoms had little impact on women's valuation of menopause (Spitzer, 1995). Role changes were common: either publicly acknowledged by taking on or expanding duties, tasks, or activities from which menstruating women were prohibited; or privately embraced by taking more time for oneself and personally imbuing this phase of life with significance.

My research resonates with other studies considering women's experience of menopause and undertaken throughout much of the world. Focusing on symptoms or a disease model of menopause greatly underestimates women's attribution of meanings to and their experiences of the change of life; instead, the menopausal transition must be considered in the broader scope of women's lives. The meanings of menopause are cultural, personal, and highly flexible. Women are capable of adapting their expectations and interpretations in new environments. Menopause is embedded in the context of a woman's life cycle, social relations, and economic situation. For foreign-born women, the process of immigration can have an impact on women's experiences of menopause; however, the nature of that impact will differ. Separation from family members, friends, and meaningful work may mean for some that this time of second youth, independence, and freedom could possibly be lost. However, balancing this loss are the benefits of living in a safe environment, providing opportunities for their children, and seeking opportunities to create and re-create meanings of menopause for themselves through introspection or prayer, or by extending their careers.

While foreign-born women may find themselves in situations where they need to adapt to novel circumstances at mid-life that differ from the menopause they might have anticipated in their native country, disparate perspectives of menopause are not limited to biomedical practitioners and foreign-born patients. Indeed, exposure to biomedicine and biomedical models of disease, including menopause, differs among the immigrant and refugee populace not only according to country of origin, but also along the lines of local geography, ethnicity, and socio-economic class. In North America, studies show that middle- and upper-class women tend to adopt the biomedical understanding of menopause more readily than working-class patients (Dickson, 1990; Martin, 1987). As I have suggested in this chapter, cultural differences pertaining to menopause emerge as much along professional and patient divides as well as along more widely acknowledged ethnic divisions. For health professionals hoping to understand the needs of mid-life women from various cultural communities, an appreciation of the dynamic cultural, economic, and personal factors that help shape all women's experience of menopause is essential.

NOTES

1. All names are pseudonyms.

REFERENCES

Amundsen, D.W., & Diers, C.J. (1970). The age of menopause in Classical Greece and Rome. *Human Biology, 42(1)*, 79–86.

———. (1973). The age of menopause in medieval Europe. *Human Biology, 45(4)*, 605–12.

Anderson, J., Blue, C., & Lau, A. (1991). Women's perspectives on chronic illness: Ethnicity, ideology and restructuring of life. *Social Science & Medicine, 32(2)*, 101–13.

Aristotle. (1763). *Aristotle's compleat masterpiece in three parts: Displaying the secrets of nature in the generation of man; treasure of health and the family physician* (29th rev.). London: Booksellers.

Avis, N., Brockwell, S., & Colvin, A. (2005). A universal menopausal syndrome? *American Journal of Medicine, 118(12B)*, 37S–46S.

Banner, L. (1992). *In full flower: Aging women, sexuality and power; A history*. New York: Alfred Knopf.

Barbe, J.W. (1993). Meno-boomers and moral guardians: An exploration of the cultural construction of menopause. In J. Callahan (Ed.), *Menopause: A midlife passage* (pp. 23–35). Bloomington: Indiana University Press.

Bruce, M., & Gottlieb, L. (1991). The meaning of time: Mohawk women at midlife. *Health Care for Women International, 12(1)*, 41–50.

Bynum, C. (1991). *Fragmentation and redemption: Essays on gender and the body in medieval religion*. New York: Zone.

Canada NewsWire. (January 23, 2003). *New survey indicates 44 per cent of Canadian women taking* HRT *have stopped* (news release). Accessed January 7, 2004, at http://www.proquest.com.proxy.bib.uottawa.ca

Chelebowski, R., Hendrix, S., Langer, R., Stefanick, M., Gass, M., Lane, D., Rodabough, R., Gilligan, M.A., Cyr, M., Thomson, C., Khandekar, J., Petrovitch, H., & McTiernan, A. (2003). Influence of estrogen plus progestin on breast cancer and mammography in healthy postmenopausal women: The women's health initiative randomized trial. *Journal of the American Medical Association, 289(24)*, 3254–63.

Csordas, T. (2002). *Body/meaning/healing.* Houndmills, UK: Palgrave Macmillan.

DeLorey, C. (1992). Differing perspectives of menopause: An attribution theory approach. In A.J. Dan & L.L. Lewis (Eds.), *Menstrual health in women's lives* (pp. 198–205). Urbana: University of Illinois Press.

Deutsch, H. (1945). *The psychology of women.* New York: Grune & Stratton.

Dickson, G. (1990). A feminist post-structuralist analysis of the knowledge of menopause. *Advancing in Nursing Science, 12(3)*, 15–31.

Diczfalusy, E. (1986). Menopause, developing countries and the 21st century. *Acta Obstetricia et Gynecologica Scandinavica, Suppl. 134*, 45–57.

Donovan, J.C. (1951). The menopausal syndrome: A study of case histories. *American Journal of Obstetrics and Gynecology, 62*, 1281–91.

Fausto-Sterling, A. (1999). Disciplining mothers: Feminism and the new reproductive technologies. In J. Price & M. Shildrick (Eds.), *Feminist theory and the body: A reader* (pp. 169–78). New York: Routledge.

Freund, P., & McGuire, M. (1995). *Health, illness and the social body: A critical sociology.* Englewood Cliffs, NJ: Prentice Hall.

Gordon, D. (1988). Tenacious assumptions in Western medicine. In M. Lock & D. Gordon (Eds.), *Biomedicine examined* (pp. 19–56). Dordrecht: Kluwer Academic.

Greenhill, M.H. (1946). The psychosomatic evaluation of the psychiatric and endocrinological factors in the menopause. *Southern Medical Journal, 39(10)*, 786–94.

Gupta, G., & Aronow, W. 2002. Hormone replacement therapy: An analysis of efficacy based on evidence. *Geriatrics, 57*, 18–24.

Humphries, K., & Gill, S. (2003). Risks and benefits of hormone replacement therapy. *Canadian Medical Association Journal, 168(8)*, 1001–10.

Jolly, E. (1997). *Surveillance and compliance.* Presentation to the Menopause in a Changing World Conference, Edmonton, AB, May 7–10.

Kaufert, P.A. (1980). The perimenopausal woman and her use of health services. *Maturitas, 2(3)*, 191–205.

Kaufert, P., & Syrotiuk, J. (1981). Symptom reporting at the menopause. *Social Science & Medicine, 15(E)*, 173–84.

Kuller, L. (2003). Hormone replacement therapy and the risk of cardiovascular disease: Implications of the results of the women's health initiative. *Artherosclerosis, Thrombosis and Vascular Biology, 23(1)*, 11–16.

Lemay, A. (2002). The relevance of the women's health initiative results on combine hormone replacement therapy in clinical practice. *Journal of Obstetrics and Gynaecology Canada, 24(9)*, 711–15.

Lock, M. (1993). *Encounters with aging: Mythologies of menopause in Japan and North America*. Berkeley: University of California Press.

Lock, M., Kaufert, P., & Gilbert, P. (1988). The cultural construction of the menopausal syndrome: The Japanese case. *Maturitas, 10*, 317–22.

Manson, J., & Martin, K. (2001). Postmenopausal hormone replacement therapy. *New England Journal of Medicine, 345(1)*, 34–40.

Martin, E. (1987). *The woman in the body: A cultural analysis of reproduction*. Boston: Beacon.

Murtagh, M., & Hepworth, J. (2003a). Feminist ethics and menopause: Autonomy and decision-making in primary medical care. *Social Science & Medicine, 56*, 1643–52.

————. (2003b) Menopause as a long-term risk to health: Implications of general practitioner accounts of prevention for women's choice and decision-making. *Sociology of Health and Illness, 25(2)*, 185–207.

North American Menopause Society (NAMS). (2002). NAMS report: Amended report from the NAMS advisory panel on postmenopausal hormone therapy. *Menopause: The Journal of the North American Menopause Society, 10(1)*, 6–12.

Odens, B.J., Boulet, M.J., Lehert, P., & Visser, A.P. (1992). Has the climacteric been medicalized? A study on the use of medication for climacteric symptoms. *Maturitas, 15*, 171–81.

Oudshoorn, N. (1994). *Beyond the natural body: The archaeology of sex hormones*. London: Routledge.

Piantadosi, S. (2003). Larger lessons from the Women's Health Initiative. *Epidemiology, 14(1)*, 6–7.

Penrose, C. (1900). *The textbook of diseases of women* (1897). Philadelphia: W.B. Saunders.

Rosenberger, N. (1986). Menopause as a symbol of anomaly: The case of Japanese women. In V. Olesen & N.F. Woods (Eds.), *Culture, society and menstruation* (pp. 15–24). New York: Hemisphere.

Rousseau, M.E. (2002). Hormone replacement therapy: Short-term versus long-term use. *Journal of Midwifery & Women's Health, 47(6)*, 461–70.

Sampselle, C., Harris, V., Harlow, S.D., & Sowers, M. (2002). Midlife development and menopause in African American and Caucasian women. *Health Care for Women International, 23*, 351–63.

Schneider, H.P.G. (2002). The view of the International Menopause Society on the Women's Health Initiative. *Climacteric, 5*, 211–16.

Shea, J. (2006). Cross-cultural comparison of women's midlife symptom-reporting: A China study. *Culture, Medicine & Psychiatry, 30*, 331–62.

Shiu-Yun, F., Anderson, D., & Courtney, M.D. (2003). Cross-cultural menopausal experience: Comparison of Australian and Taiwanese women. *Nursing & Health Sciences, 5*, 77–84.

Smith-Rosenberg, C. (1985). *Disorderly conduct: Visions of gender in Victorian America*. New York: Alfred A. Knopf.

Society of Obstetricians and Gynaecologists of Canada (SOGC). (2003). *Appendix: Revisions to recommendations; Canadian consensus on menopause and osteoporosis*. Accessed May 30, 2003, from the Society of Obstetricians and Gynaecologists of Canada website at http://www.sogc.org/guidelines/public/108E-CONS2-Sep-Dec2001.pdf

——. (2006). *The journalists' menopause handbook: A companion guide to the Society of Obstetricians and Gynaecologists of Canada menopause consensus report*. Ottawa: Society of Obstetricians and Gynaecologists of Canada.

Spitzer, D.L. (1995). More than the change: Diversity and flexibility in menopausal experiences. In L. Taetzsch (Ed.), *Hot flashes: Women writers on the change of life* (pp. 115–31). New York: Faber & Faber.

——. (2003). Panic and panaceas: Hormone replacement therapy and the menopausal syndrome. *Atlantis: A Women's Studies Journal, 27(2)*, 6–13.

——. (2007). Immigrant and refugee women: Re-creating meaning in trans-national context. *Anthropology in Action, 14(1 & 2)*, 52–62.

——. (2009). Crossing cultural and bodily boundaries of migration and menopause. In L. Hernandez & S. Krajewski (Eds.), *Crossing Cultural Boundaries* (pp. 148–58). Cambridge, UK: Cambridge Scholars Publishing.

Thomas, T.G. (1880). *A practical treatise on the diseases of women*. Philadelphia: Henry C. Lea.

U.S. Preventative Services Task Force (USPSTF). (2003). Postmenopausal hormone replacement therapy for the primary prevention of chronic conditions: Recommendations and rationale. *American Family Physician, 67(2)*, 358–64.

Watson, L.C., & Watson-Franke, M.-B. (1985). *Interpreting life histories: An anthropological inquiry*. New Brunswick, NJ: Rutgers University Press.

Wilbush, J. (1980). Historical Perspective: Tilt, E.J. and the change of life (1857)—The only work on the subject in the English language. *Maturitas, 2(4)*, 259–67.

——. (1986). The climacteric syndrome: Historical perspectives. In M. Notelovitz & P. Van Keep (Eds.), *The climacteric in perspective: Proceedings of the fourth international congress on the menopause* (pp. 121–29). Lancaster: MTP Press.

Women's Health Initiative Investigators Writing Group (WHI). (2002). Risks and benefits of estrogen plus progestin in healthy postmenopausal women: Principal results from the women's health initiative randomized controlled trial. *Journal of the American Medical Association, 288(3)*, 321–33.

TWELVE

HEALTH AND HEALTH CARE UTILIZATION PATTERNS OF VISIBLE MINORITY SENIORS IN CANADA

Juhee Vajracharya Suwal PhD

INTRODUCTION

Peoples' perception of health may influence their health care utilization pattern, and visible minority immigrants are no exception. Coming to a new country and facing various challenges such as adjusting to a different culture, language barriers, economic disadvantage, less social support, lack of easy access to transportation, and lack of general and health information may make immigrants, especially senior immigrants belonging to a visible minority group, vulnerable to ill health. For these same reasons, they may be reluctant to use available health services. Identifying health services utilization behaviours and the health status of visible minority seniors will help policy planners understand the health and social needs of this particular group, and thus will eventually help planners better provide culturally appropriate health services and minimize the cost of health care at the same time. The health status and health care use of senior visible minority groups have not received much attention despite their growing number in Canada. This study compares the health status of visible minority and White seniors in Canada, and analyzes the relationship between visible minority seniors' health services use and factors that may affect the use and non-use of available services.

Current Situation of Visible Minority Seniors in Canada

Visible minorities are defined by the *Employment Equity Act* as "persons, other than Aboriginal peoples, who are non-Caucasian in race or non-White in colour" (Statistics Canada, 2001a). Until the 1950s, most immigrants to Canada were from European countries, whereas the trend has shifted to visible minorities since 1997 (Hyman, 2001). According to the 2001 census, 13.44% of Canada's population of 29,639,030 belong to visible minority groups. Of these visible minorities, 6.5% were seniors (Statistics Canada, 2001b). The census records also show that most members of visible minority groups (54.4%) live in Ontario, 21% live in British Columbia, 12.5% in Quebec, and 8.3% in Alberta; the lowest number (N = 210) live in Nunavut. Of all the visible minorities in the 2001 census, 70% were born outside of Canada; Chinese accounted for 26% and South Asians 23% (Statistics Canada, 2005). Canada's visible minority population is expected to increase to 7.1 million in 2026 from 2.7 million in 1996. Between 1996 and 2001, the rate of growth of visible minorities was noticeably faster than that of the total population of Canada—25% for visible minorities as compared to 4% for the whole population (National Advisory Council on Aging, 2005).

The population distribution of elderly immigrants will eventually change with a higher proportion of visible minority seniors than other immigrant seniors as a result of the continuous increase in visible minority immigrants. This trend will grow much faster as the visible minority baby boomers age. There were about 20% visible minorities in the age group 45–64 in the 2001 census (Statistics Canada, 2001b) who were about to become seniors in 2002 or in the coming years. Thus the planners in Canada will have to meet the health and social needs of the elderly as well as understand the socio-cultural norms of health concepts of visible minority groups.

Some social scientists argue that the elderly among visible minorities may be victims of so-called "double jeopardy," being old and belonging to a marginalized group (Dowd & Bengtson, 1978). However, other researchers have shown that this hypothesis is weak or that the difference in indicators between White and minority seniors narrows with age (Penning, 1983;

Rosenthal, 1983; Chan, 1983; Rosenthal, 1986). Furthermore, researchers also caution us to look at different socio-economic variables, such as education and income of visible minority groups, to investigate whether multiple or double jeopardy affects only those with low education levels and low income, and whether the effect is thus not due to belonging to a visible minority group (Durst, 2005). This study will shed light on some of these issues with empirical evidence using the current status of health and health care utilization of visible minority seniors in Canada.

Perceptions on Health

It is a well-established fact that the perception of health among different cultural groups around the world varies. As Lai, Tsang, Chappell, Lai, and Chau (2003) found, such perceptions vary even among the Chinese, depending on their country of origin. Immigrants may adhere to their traditional social norms and health perceptions in their new country. Age-related illness such as dementia is taken as a natural process of aging among the Vietnamese and the Hawaiians living in the United States, for example (Braun & Browne, 1998). Braun and Browne (1998) discussed cases among Chinese, Japanese, and Filipino immigrants, who believed in links between illnesses and wrongful acts in previous lives. Another study found that Chinese Americans hid persons with disability while Korean immigrants in that study group preferred to seek informal and formal help only if provided by Koreans (McCallion, Janicki, & Grant-Griffin, 1997). Even the choice of words to denote certain "diseases" should be selected carefully while dealing with seniors from visible minority groups. For example, mental health is a taboo subject among the elderly Chinese, and they may identify mental health "by referring to it as 'mood,' a word with fewer stigmas attached" (Lai, 2003).

Health Status of Immigrants

There have been a considerable number of research findings on the "healthy immigrant effect" in Canada recently. Normally, immigrants are healthy when they enter Canada, probably because of the health screening required in the immigration process (Dunn & Dyck, 2000). After being in Canada for more than ten years, immigrants' health status seems to converge with that of Canadians (Chen, Ng, & Wilkins, 1996; Newbold & Danforth, 2003; Dunn & Dyck, 2004; McDonald, Clarke, McLeary, George, & Marziali, 2006). By using the 2001 Canadian Community Health Survey,

Perez (2002) showed that Canadian immigrants had better health than non-immigrants in terms of chronic conditions as well. In addition, the results also revealed that recently arrived males had healthier heart disease outcomes than non-immigrants and that recently arrived female immigrants had fewer cancer problems than their non-immigrant counterparts. Similarly, Ali (2002) found that recent immigrants and immigrants from Asia and Africa had lower rates of depression and alcohol dependence than the Canadian-born population even after adjustment for age, gender, marital status, income, and education. This result held true despite immigrants' language barriers, higher unemployment rates, and lower sense of belonging to the local community. Furthermore, older ethnic minority persons, most of whom had immigrated to Canada "ten years or more" earlier, had poorer health status in comparison to the ethnic majority group (McDonald, Clarke, McLeary, George, & Marziali, 2006).

Ng, Wilkins, Gendron, and Berthelot (2005) conducted a longitudinal study of non-European and European immigrants' health versus "other" Canadians' health by using all five cycles of National Population Health Survey data. Both recent and long-term (immigrated before 1981) non-European immigrants were twice as likely to report their health as poor or fair in 2002–2003, compared to Canadian-born individuals. However, these same non-European immigrants reported their health as excellent or very good in 1994–1995. As a result of deteriorating health, non-European immigrants also visited medical doctors more often than other Canadians in 2002–2003. Stress of immigration and gain in weight because of lack of physical activity were also found. Nonetheless, literature on senior immigrants' health status has mixed findings. Newbold and Filice (2006) found both immigrant and non-immigrant seniors rank their health in a similar manner. In contrast, Lai et al. (2003) found that Chinese seniors' health was poorer than those of the "other" population in Canada. The cultural norms and health care services use of a specific group among immigrants, perhaps, made the difference. This study will examine whether the healthy immigrant effect found among immigrants in Canada holds true in the case of senior visible minority population.

Health Services Utilization and Access to Services

If individuals perceive their health condition as excellent, they may not seek medical help. Similarly, financial situations, language barriers, educational background, and other circumstantial factors may have an impact on an individual's choice to seek preventative medical help. It is important to keep in mind that the perception of health and mental health of various cultures comes to play a big role in seeking any kind of medical help. Generally speaking, seniors may be physically challenged compared to younger people, and thus may tend to use health care more often. One recent study found that almost 90% of Canadian seniors consulted a family doctor, 14% were hospitalized, and 15% received home care in a year (Rotermann, 2006). The main reason for health care use by seniors was a chronic health condition. Not surprisingly, cultural factors were found to contribute to the health care utilization differential among seniors belonging to Asian Pacific Islander groups in the United States (Tanjasiri, Wallace, & Shibata, 1995). The elderly in this group delayed in seeking care, were confused in making appointments, had a language barrier, felt embarrassed and afraid while attempting to describe symptoms, and were confused, afraid, or angered at professional advice.

One recent Canadian study found that although visible minorities in general were more likely than White Canadians to have had contact with a general practitioner and were less likely to have contact with specialists, specific subgroups of visible minorities—such as the Japanese and the Koreans—used both general practitioners and specialists less frequently than their White counterparts (Quan et al., 2006). However, the empirical study by Jenkins, Le, Mcphee, Stewart, and Ha (1996) on Vietnamese immigrants in California demonstrated that it was accessibility to the health care system rather than cultural health beliefs and practices that determined preventive health care utilization among this group. Lai et al. (2003) found that Chinese seniors in Canada had a low level of home support services use compared to the general population despite the former group's poorer health status. They also found that Chinese seniors did not seek help from mental health care providers despite having poorer mental health than the general population.

Similar to other immigrants, visible minority immigrants, especially seniors, leave behind their close friends and relatives, a prestigious living style, name, and/or fame to come to Canada to join their children. For visible minority immigrant seniors in Canada, a feeling of loneliness and depression (Kinch & Jakubec, 2004; Acharya, 2004) and being in "golden prison" at home (Durst, 2005) are not uncommon; these feelings have been discussed in a number of qualitative and quantitative studies. Considering these facts, living in Canada for a long period may mean deterioration in health for these seniors. Given other disadvantages they may face, such as discrimination (Neufeld, Harrison, Stewart, Hughes, & Spitzer, 2002; Ng, Northcott, & Abu-Laban, 2004) and low income (Harvey, Siu, & Reil, 1999), they may also become victims of double or multiple jeopardy. The purpose of this study is to unveil the demographic, socio-economic and health status, lifestyle, and health care service utilization patterns of visible minority seniors versus White seniors based on empirical analysis, with the objectives of: (a) examining the healthy immigrant effect, (b) revisiting the double/multiple jeopardy thesis, and (c) providing valuable policy implications for health and social policy planners in Canada.

METHODS

The data source for this study was the Public Use Microdata File (PUMF) of the Canadian Community Health Survey Cycle 3.1 conducted in year 2005. This PUMF contains the regional, provincial, and national information on health services, health status, and health issues important to Canadians and disseminated to the public (Statistics Canada, 2006). The sample data contained 132,221 respondents aged 12 years and older. A Random Digit Dialing sampling frame was used to select the household sample for this survey. Individuals living on Indian Reserves and on Crown Lands, institutional residents, full-time members of the Canadian Forces, and residents of certain remote regions were excluded from the survey. The response rate was 78.9% (Statistics Canada, 2006).

For the current study, visible minorities and Whites aged 65 and over were selected for analysis, using the "cultural/racial" question. Unfortunately, cultural/ethnic groups were not specified by each cultural group in the PUMF data as they were in the original data file. The total sub-sample turned out to be 19,146 cases, of which 1,625 seniors belonged to visible minority groups (8.5%) and 16,781 were White (87.6%); the rest (3.9%, N = 739) did not specify their cultural status. The data were analyzed by using Pearson's chi-square test. The variables selected for analysis were cultural identity (visible minority seniors versus Whites); demographic and socio-economic (gender, job status, education level, language proficiency, living arrangement, household size, personal income, length of stay in Canada); health status (chronic condition, arthritis/rheumatism, high blood pressure, heart disease); perceived health and perceived mental health; health care services utilization (has regular medical doctor, number of visits to a doctor, reasons for not having a regular doctor, consulted alternate health care provider, had flu shot, had eyes examined, visited dentist, overnight patient, required home care provided by the government, required home care not covered by the government). Comparative analyses were performed by cultural/racial group (visible minority or White) and by gender, education, income, language proficiency, and years of stay in Canada among visible minority seniors.

RESULTS

Demographic Characteristics

Among the visible minority seniors, 81.0% were immigrants, whereas 21.5% of White seniors were immigrants. Of those visible minority senior immigrants, 88.2% had lived in Canada for ten or more years and the rest less than ten years, whereas almost all (99.0%, N = 3,564) White seniors who self-identified as immigrants had lived in Canada for ten or more years (table 1). In both visible minority and Whites groups, female seniors were represented more than males. Some visible minority and White seniors were still working full-time or part-time. Most visible minority seniors had either "less than secondary" education or were "post-secondary" graduates, similar to those belonging to the White group. Although a large percentage of visible minorities reported that they spoke either English or French or both, with or without other languages, 27.2% (N = 440) of these seniors did not speak either of the official languages.

The "living arrangement" and "household size" results from table 1 confirm that one-third of visible minority seniors lived in "other" arrangements rather than alone or with spouse, or in parent-spouse-child or parent-child arrangements, possibly in large households with four or more persons. Half as many visible minority seniors as Whites lived alone, and two-thirds as many lived with a spouse only, compared to Whites. Personal income showed that 61% of visible minority elderly earned below $15,000 or none at all, almost double the proportion of low-income Whites.

Health Characteristics

A large proportion from both groups (about 90%) had a chronic health condition. Relative to visible minorities, a significantly higher proportion of White seniors had arthritis or rheumatism and heart disease. A significantly higher proportion of visible minority elderly were suffering from high blood pressure relative to Whites (table 1).

Perceived Health Status

About one-third of visible minority elderly said their health was in excellent or very good condition (table 2). About the same proportions indicated their health as good and as fair or poor. A higher percentage of White seniors (40.6%) than visible minorities confirmed their health as excellent or very good. Most seniors from both groups (62% of visible minority and 69.5% of White seniors) perceived their mental health to be excellent or very good. Relative to general health, substantially low percentages from both groups expressed their mental health as fair or poor. However, a higher percentage of visible minority seniors (8.4%) reported their mental health as fair or poor compared to Whites (4.7%).

Health Services Utilization

Most seniors from both groups had a regular doctor: 96.3% of visible minority versus 95.2% of White respondents (table 2). Nevertheless, the former group visited their doctors more often than their White counterparts. A significantly higher proportion of White seniors reported that the doctor they saw had either left or retired, among other reasons for not having a doctor. About 10.7% of visible minorities and 6.3% of Whites consulted alternate health care providers.

A significantly higher proportion of White seniors were overnight patients compared to their visible minority counterparts. A higher proportion of White seniors than visible minority seniors also needed home care provided by the government as well as that not covered by the government. The differentials between the groups of those who responded to flu-shot questions and those who responded to eye-examination questions were narrow. Nonetheless, the proportion of visible minority elderly who visited the dentist less than a year ago was fairly low (48.5%) relative to Whites (56.1%).

The lifestyle factor measured by smoking and drinking was also examined for both groups. Most seniors from both groups were non-smokers. Compared to visible minority seniors, almost double the proportion (9.0%) of White seniors smoked daily. More than one-half of White seniors were regular drinkers in comparison to one-third of visible minorities. Among the visible minority elderly, 29% never drank liquor as opposed to 7.9% Whites. Almost the same proportion of seniors from both groups (about 7%) also indicated unmet health care needs.

Perceived Health Within Visible Minority Group by Different Characteristics

A lower percentage of female visible minority seniors indicated both their general health (30.5%) and mental health (61.4%) as excellent or very good compared to males (38.3% and 64.6% respectively) (table 3). Within the three education levels, the highest proportion of visible minority seniors with university degree (40.5%) reported having an excellent or very good health and the lowest proportion (20.8%) as fair or poor health (table 3). In contrast, most of those who had less than high school education (40.9%) reported their health as fair or poor. Reports on mental health are consistent across every education level, the highest proportions reporting as excellent or very good and the lowest proportions as fair or poor in each category of education. However, visible minority seniors with a university degree mostly (75.1%) reported having excellent or very good mental health, with few (3.3%) reporting fair or poor mental health.

The haves and have-nots among the visible minority seniors reported very different levels of self-perceived health, especially self-perceived mental health: more than one-third of those with less than $30,000 annual income reported their health as fair or poor, compared to one-tenth of those whose income was $30,000 or more. Less than 27.5% of low-income seniors perceived their health to be excellent or very good relative to 58.4% of high-income seniors. Similarly, 59.3% of seniors with low income perceived their mental health as excellent or very good, whereas 80.6% of seniors belonging to the high-income group perceived the same.

Language Proficiency

The percentages of those who perceived their health, especially mental health, as excellent or very good were significantly lower for those who could not converse in English or French as opposed to those who could converse in one of the official languages (table 3). The percentages of seniors who reported their health and mental health as fair or poor were significantly higher if they could not converse in English or French than those who could converse in one of the official languages. A significantly higher percentage of visible minority seniors who could not converse in English or French had a regular medical doctor, visited a doctor more than seven times a year, consulted an alternate health care provider, and had a flu shot within the past year compared to those who could converse in one of the official languages (table 4). A significantly lower percentage of visible minority seniors who could not speak either of the official languages had had their eyes examined and visited a dentist within the past year, compared to those who could speak English or French.

Apart from these findings, chronic conditions and health services utilization of visible minority seniors by gender and income were also examined. A higher percentage of female visible minority seniors reported having a chronic condition and a regular doctor than their male counterparts. However, a higher percentage of male visible minority seniors saw their doctors more than 19 times compared to females. Having a flu shot and eye examination were not very different for males versus females. A moderately higher percentage of females visited a dentist within the past year than their male counterparts.

A remarkably high percentage of visible minority seniors from low-income group saw the doctor more than 7 times and as high as 19 times or more, compared with those from the high-income group. Interestingly, a significantly higher percentage from the low-income group had a flu shot in the past year compared to those in the high-income group. In contrast, only 55.8% of those coming from the low-income group had visited a dentist in the past year, in comparison to 86% from the higher income group.

Healthy Immigrant Effect

Although there was some indication that recent arrivals among visible minority seniors had better health and mental health compared to those who had been to Canada for ten years or more, length-of-stay in Canada results were not significant (table 3). A remarkably higher percentage (91.0%) of earlier arrivals reported having a chronic illness as opposed to 74.5% of recent arrivals (table 4). Similarly, 34.8% of earlier arrivals saw the doctor more than six times a year, whereas 24.3% recent arrivals reported the same. Almost the same percentage (about 58.0%) of both early and recent arrivals visited a dentist in the past year.

DISCUSSION

Unlike the findings of Newbold and Filice (2006), in which native- and foreign-born people aged 55 and over ranked their health in a similar manner, we found differences in perceived health, perceived mental health, chronic conditions, lifestyle, and health care service use between visible minority and White seniors in Canada. We also found differences in these factors by gender, education levels, language proficiency, income levels, and length of stay in Canada within the visible minority group.

What is also clear from this study is that more White seniors live alone, and they make more money than their visible minority counterparts. One-third of visible minority seniors live in large households with four or more people. This may be because most seniors from visible minority backgrounds come to Canada to look after their grandchildren (National Advisory Council on Aging, 2005) or to join their adult children (Behjati-Sabet & Chambers, 2005; Dinh, Ganesan, & Waxler-Morrison, 2005). This could also be one of the reasons why their individual income is less than that of White seniors.

It is a matter of concern that a lower percentage of visible minority seniors than Whites perceive their health and mental health as excellent or very good, and that a higher percentage of visible minority seniors report their health and mental health as fair or poor. Regardless of race or ethnicity, most seniors had some kind of chronic health problem. The chronic conditions could be the reason why such a high percentage of seniors from both groups had a regular medical doctor. Given the high prevalence of chronic illnesses reported by seniors, the remarkable proportion having fair or poor health, and their high utilization of health care facilities, increased health care costs could be expected in the coming years. High blood pressure was more prevalent among visible minority elderly, but the direction of prevalence changes favouring them over the Whites in such chronic conditions as heart disease and arthritis/rheumatism.

The healthy immigrant effect that most researchers have found was not fully confirmed in the case of visible minority seniors. However, there was a suggestion of healthy immigrant effect for visible minority seniors in relation to their chronic condition and doctor's visits.

While comparing the health and health care services utilization pattern, we had an opportunity to revisit the "double jeopardy/multiple jeopardy" thesis for visible minority seniors. There were some suggestions that visible minority seniors may have been disadvantaged to some extent because of their minority status apart from belonging to a low-income group. Language proficiency proved to be very important in having excellent health, especially mental health. More importantly, the findings also suggest that it is their lack of language proficiency that poses a barrier to health care services use, such as seeking eye and dental care. Language proficiency was also related to fewer visits to a doctor. The language barrier, of course, is connected to their status as minority senior immigrants.

Visible minority seniors' lower utilization of health care services such as eye examinations, dentistry, being an overnight hospital patient, and having government-provided home care may also depend on culture, perception of health, and lifestyle, along with language barriers and personal income. A low percentage of visible minority seniors reporting excellent or very good health may be a result of the types of food they consume in Canada, their economic condition, the difficulty of coping with the harsh winter (Dinh et al., 2005), the stress of leaving their friends and relatives back home to come to a new place and unfamiliar culture, and loss of social status. Similarly, visible minority seniors' higher number of visits to the doctor could be the outcome of their poor health.

Researchers acknowledge the fact that the study of immigrants is complex (Durst, 2005), and the complexity may become greater when the study is that of senior visible minority immigrants for several reasons. First, some visible minority seniors were born in Canada or had resided in Canada for decades, obviously with more acculturation, while others were recent immigrants (possibly facing various challenges). Second, visible minority groups have complex cultures and different norms related to aging and health compared to other immigrants. Third, despite their growing numbers in Canada, relatively little research has been conducted on this segment of the population, and thus detailed medical and health-related information about this population has not been known.

From the findings of this study, there arise a number of medical and health-related research questions that are worth exploring in the future. A relationship between the higher percentage of visible minority seniors suffering from high blood pressure and the stress related to large family households, the depression of being left alone with small children or infants in the house, and/or loneliness (while sons, daughters, and daughters-in-law are at work) may unveil a number of answers for these seniors' health outcomes and challenges they face. Similarly, a relationship between visible minority seniors' high blood pressure and their changed lifestyle and/or changed diet in Canada could be worth examining. Another interesting study could be to investigate the factors influencing the use of alternate health care providers. What could be done to improve the double or multiple jeopardy situation of senior visible minority population in Canada may be yet another research question for future researchers to explore.

LIMITATIONS

A larger sample size and including specific visible minority groups in the PUMF data would be useful for researchers interested in these groups. Not all visible minority groups have similar cultures, neither do they come to Canada with similar reasons for migration, nor do they have homogenous perceptions of health and aging. A multiple regression analysis may reveal relationships between predictor variables selected and visible minority seniors' health and health care utilization outcomes. Apart from empirical analysis, qualitative research may expose a number of hidden causes of deterioration of health and mental health over time for visible minority seniors in Canada.

CONCLUSION

Given that most (75%) of the recent immigrants to Canada belong to a visible minority group (Ng, Wilkins, Gendron, & Berthelot, 2005), studies of visible minority seniors, their health, mental health, and health care use become more important as their numbers keep growing. Furthermore, general health and mental health become fragile as people age, needing more health care services use in the future. Thus, keeping track of visible minority seniors' health and mental health, use of health care services, and access to preventative health services will help Canadian health policy planners tremendously in the process of health provision, health-related infrastructure building, and training of health professionals in dealing with culturally sensitive "elderly health" related issues, especially focused on visible minorities. Such processes will eventually be beneficial in maintaining the health of visible minority seniors for a healthier Canada, while at the same time in reducing health care costs.

AUTHOR'S NOTE

The author is grateful to Chuck Humphrey of the data library, University of Alberta for providing the Canadian Community Health Survey, 2005 PUMF data and to Dr. Andrew Cave of the Department of Family Medicine, University of Alberta, for his suggestions on an earlier version of this article.

REFERENCES

Acharya, M.P. (2004). *Constructing the meaning of "mental distress": Coping strategies of elderly East Indian immigrant women in Alberta*. PHD thesis, Department of Sociology, University of Alberta, Edmonton, AB, Canada.

Ali, J. (2002,). Mental health of Canada's immigrants (catalogue no. 82-003). *Supplement to Health Reports, 13*. Ottawa: Statistics Canada.

Behjati-Sabet, A., & Chambers, N.A. (2005). People of Iranian descent. In N. Waxler-Morrison, J.M. Anderson, E. Richardson, & N.A. Chambers (Eds.), *Cross-cultural caring: A handbook for health professionals* (pp. 127–61). Vancouver: UBC Press.

Braun, K.L., & Browne, C.V. (1998). Perceptions of dementia, caregiving, and help seeking among Asian and Pacific Islander Americans. *Health & Social Work, 23(4)*, 262–74.

Chan, K.B. (1983). Coping with aging and managing self-identity: The social world of the elderly Chinese women. *Canadian Ethnic Studies, 15(3)*, 36–50.

Chen, J., Ng, E., & Wilkins, R. (1996). The health of Canada's immigrants in 1994–95. *Health Reports, 7(4)*, 33–45.

Dinh, D.K., Ganesan, S., & Waxler-Morrison, N. (2005). People of Vietnamese descent. In N. Waxler-Morrison, J.M. Anderson, E. Richardson, & N.A. Chambers (Eds.), *Cross-cultural caring: A handbook for health professionals* (pp. 247–87). Vancouver: UBC Press.

Dowd, J.J., & Bengtson, V.L. (1978). Aging in minority populations: An examination of the double jeopardy hypothesis. *Journal of Gerontology, 33(3)*, 427–36.

Dunn, J.R., & Dyck, I. (2000). Social determinants of health in Canada's immigrant population: Results from the National Population Health Survey. *Social Science & Medicine, 51*, 1573–93.

Durst, D. (2005). *Aging amongst immigrant in Canada: Policy and planning implications*. Paper presented at the 12th Biennial Canadian Social Welfare Policy Conference: Forging Social Futures, Fredericton, NB.

Harvey, E.B., Siu, B., & Reil, K.D.V. (1999). Ethno-cultural groups, period of immigration and socioeconomic situations. *Canadian Ethnic Studies, 31(3)*, 95–103.

Hyman, I. (2001). *Immigration and health* (No. 01–05). Health Policy Workshop Paper Series. Ottawa: Health Canada.

Jenkins, C.N.H., Le, T., Mcphee, S.J., Stewart, S., & Ha, N.T. (1996). Health care access and preventative care among Vietnamese immigrants: Do traditional beliefs and practices pose barriers? *Social Science & Medicine, 43(7)*, 1049–56.

Kinch, J.L., & Jakubec, S. (2004). "Multiple margins" (being older, a woman, or a visible minority) constrained older women's access to Canadian health care. *Canadian Journal of Nursing Research, 36*, 90–108.

Lai, D.W.L. (2003). Measuring depression of elderly Chinese Americans: A replication study. *Home Health Care Services Quarterly, 22(2)*, 69–85.

Lai, D.W.L., Tsang, K.T., Chappell, N.L., Lai, D.C.Y., & Chau, S.B.Y. (2003). *Health and well being of older Chinese in Canada*. Calgary: Centre on Aging, Faculty of Social Work, University of Calgary.

McCallion, P., Janicki, M., & Grant-Griffin, L. (1997). Exploring the impact of culture and acculturation on older families caregiving for persons with developmental disabilities. *Family Relations, 46(4)*, 347–57.

McDonald, L., Clarke, D., McLeary, L., George, U., & Marziali, E. (2006). *Health disparities in older visible minorities in Canada.* Paper presented at the Meeting the Challenge: Research in and with Diverse Communities Conference, Society for Social Work and Research, January 2006, San Antonio, TX.

National Advisory Council on Aging. (2005). *Seniors on the margin: Seniors from ethno-cultural minorities.* Ottawa: National Advisory Council on Aging.

Neufeld, A., Harrison, M.J., Stewart, M.J., Hughes, K.D., & Spitzer, D. (2002). Immigrant women: Making connections to community resources for support in family caregiving. *Qualitative Health Research, 12(6)*, 751–68.

Newbold, B.K., & Filice, J.K. (2006). Health status of older immigrants to Canada. *Canadian Journal on Aging, 25(3)*, 305–19.

Newbold, B.K., & Danforth, J. (2003). Health status and Canada's immigrant population. *Social Science & Medicine, 57*, 1981–95.

Ng, C.F., Northcott, H.C., & Abu-Laban, S.M. (2004). *The experiences of South Asian immigrant seniors living in Edmonton, Alberta: Report to the community.* Edmonton: Alberta Centre on Aging, University of Alberta.

Ng, E., Wilkins, R., Gendron, F., & Berthelot, J. (2005). *Dynamics of immigrants' health in Canada: Evidence from the National Population Health Survey* (catalogue no. 82-618-MWE2005002). Ottawa: Statistics Canada.

Penning, M.J. (1983). Multiple jeopardy: Age sex, and ethnic variations. *Canadian Ethnic Studies, 15(3)*, 81–105.

Perez, C.E. (2002). Health status and health behaviour among immigrants (Catalogue no. 82-003). *Supplements to Health Reports, 13.* Ottawa: Statistics Canada.

Quan, H., Fong, A., De Coster, C., Wang, J., Musto, R., Noseworthy, T.W., & Ghali, W.A. (2006). Variation in health services utilization among ethnic populations. *Canadian Medical Association Journal, 174(6)*, 787–91.

Rosenthal, C.J. (1983). Aging, ethnicity and the family: Beyond the modernization thesis. *Canadian Ethnic Studies, 15(3)*, 1–16.

————. (1986). Family supports in later life: Does ethnicity make a difference? *Gerontologist, 26(1)*, 19–24.

Rotermann, M. (2006). Seniors' health care use (Catalogue no. 82-003). *Supplement to Health Reports, 16.* Ottawa: Statistics Canada.

Statistics Canada. (2001a). Definition: Visible minority population by age, provinces and territories (2001 Census). Accessed November 27, 2007, at http://www.statcan.ca/english/Pgdb/defdemo50a.htm

————. (2001b). Visible minority population by age (2001 Census). Accessed December 3, 2006, at http://www.statcan.ca/english/Pgdb/demo50a.htm

————. (2005). Study: Canada's visible minority population in 2017. *Daily*, March 22. Accessed November 27, 2007, at http://www.statcan.ca/Daily/English/050322/d050322b.htm

————. (2006). *Canadian Community Health Survey (CCHS) Cycle 3.1, 2005; Public Use Microdata File (PUMF) Use Guide*. Ottawa: Statistics Canada.

Tanjasiri, S.P., Wallace, S.P., & Shibata, K. (1995). Picture imperfect: Hidden problems among Asian Pacific Islander elderly. *Gerontologist, 35(6)*, 753–60.

TABLE 1: *Demographics of Visible Minority and White Seniors, 2005*

Indicators	Seniors aged 65 and over		
	Visible minorities N (%)	Whites N (%)	p-value
Demographics			
Status: Immigrant	1,299 (81.0)	3,601 (21.5)	0.000
Length of stay in Canada:			
0–9 years	153 (11.8)	37 (1.0)	0.000
10 years or more	1,146 (88.2)	3,564 (99.0)	
Gender:			
Male	706 (43.4)	7,472 (44.5)	0.209
Female	919 (56.6)	9,310 (55.5)	
Job:			
Full-time	70 (61.4)	744 (56.9)	0.354
Part-time	44 (38.6)	563 (43.1)	
Education:			
Less than secondary	705 (44.2)	6,973 (42.2)	
Secondary grad/other post-secondary	264 (14.3)	3,185 (19.3)	0.008
Post-secondary graduates	627 (39.3)	6,352 (38.5)	
Language (can converse):			
English/French	1,179 (73.8)	16,536 (98.6)	0.000
No English/French	440 (27.2)	224 (1.4)	
Living arrangement:			
Unattached/alone	253 (15.6)	5,078 (30.3)	
With spouse/partner	545 (33.7)	8,961 (53.5)	
Parent, spouse, child	207 (12.8)	893 (5.3)	0.000
Parent and child	63 (3.9)	634 (3.8)	
Other	550 (34.0)	1,176 (7.1)	
Household size:			
1 person	253 (15.6)	5,078 (30.3)	
2 persons	642 (39.5)	9,888 (58.9)	0.000
3 or more persons	730 (45.0)	2,327 (10.8)	
Personal income:			
< 15,000	760 (61.4)	4,384 (32.9)	
15,000–49,000	397 (32.1)	7,561 (56.6)	0.000
50,000 and over	80 (6.4)	1,409 (10.6)	
Health Characteristics			
Has chronic condition (yes)	1,459 (89.8)	15,259 (91.1)	0.055
Has arthritis/rheumatism (yes)	609 (37.6)	7,853 (46.9)	0.000
Has high blood pressure (yes)	781 (48.1)	7,375 (44.0)	0.001
Has heart disease (yes)	204 (12.6)	3,301 (19.7)	0.000
Total N	1,625	16,781	

Source: Computed from the Canadian Community Health Survey, Cycle 3.1, Public Use Microdata File.

Note: Percentages in each cell show those who responded to that particular question.

TABLE 2: *Health Care Utilization and Health of Visible Minorities and Whites, 2005*

Indicators	Seniors aged 65 and over		
	Visible minorities N (%)	Whites N (%)	p-value
Perceived Health			
Self-perceived health:			
Excellent/very good	549 (33.8)	6,785 (40.6)	0.000
Good	565 (34.9)	5,679 (33.9)	
Fair/poor	507 (31.3)	4,278 (25.6)	
Self-perceived mental health:			
Excellent/very good	891 (62.8)	11,005 (69.5)	0.000
Good	408 (28.8)	4,075 (25.7)	
Fair/poor	119 (8.4)	747 (4.7)	
Health Services Utilization			
Has regular medical doctor (yes)	1,565 (96.3)	15,973 (95.2)	0.025
Reasons for not having a regular doctor:			
No doctor available	— (—)	108 (13.4)	0.113
Not taking new patients	— (—)	117 (14.6)	0.522
Not tried to contact one	22 (36.7)	217 (27.0)	0.074
Doctor has left/retired	— (—)	266 (33.1)	0.002
Other	15 (25.0)	208 (25.9)	0.510
Number of visits to a doctor:			
1–6 times	1,013 (67.7)	11,175 (73.6)	0.000
7 times or more	484 (32.3)	4,005 (26.4)	
Consulted alternate health provider (yes)	174 (10.7)	1,060 (6.3)	0.000
Last time had flu shot:			
< 1 year	967 (88.1)	11,314 (88.6)	0.021
1–2 years	54 (4.9)	439 (3.4)	
2 years or more	76 (6.9)	1,022 (8.0)	
Last time eyes examined:			
< 1 year	492 (66.8)	4,090 (69.0)	0.070
1–2 years	130 (17.7)	964 (16.3)	
2 years or more	112 (15.3)	841 (14.2)	
Last time visited dentist:			
< 1 year	364 (48.5)	3,709 (56.1)	0.000
1–2 years	57 (7.6)	497 (7.5)	
2 years or more	296 (39.4)	2,308 (34.9)	
never	34 (4.5)	96 (1.5)	
Overnight patient (yes)	166 (10.4)	2,390 (14.3)	0.000
Required home care provided by govt. (yes)	92 (5.7)	1,597 (9.5)	0.000
Required home care not covered by govt. (yes)	138 (8.5)	1,549 (9.2)	0.325
Total N	1,625	16,781	

Source: Computed from Canadian Community Health Survey, Cycle 3.1, Public Use Microdata File.

Note: Percentages in each cell show those who responded to that particular question.

TABLE 3: *Perceived Health and Mental Health of Visible Minorities by Gender, Education, and Income, 2005*

Indicators	Perceived health (visible minority seniors)		
	Excellent/ very good	Good	Fair/poor
Gender:			
Male	269 (38.3)	239 (34.0)	195 (27.7)
Female	280 (30.5)	356 (35.5)	312 (34.0)
Education:*			
Less than high school	202 (28.6)	215 (30.5)	288 (40.9)
High school + some university	86 (32.6)	98 (37.1)	80 (30.3)
University graduates	253 (40.5)	241 (38.6)	210 (20.8)
Personal income:*			
Less than $30,000	290 (27.5)	397 (37.7)	366 (34.8)
$30,000 and over	108 (58.4)	58 (31.4)	19 (10.3)
Language proficiency:			
English/French	427 (36.3)	401 (34.1)	347 (29.5)
No English/French	119 (27.0)	164 (37.2)	158 (35.8)
Years of stay in Canada:			
< 10 years	54 (35.5)	59 (38.3)	39 (25.7)
10+ years	373 (32.5)	394 (34.4)	379 (33.1)

Indicators	Perceived mental health (visible minority seniors)		
	Excellent/ very good	Good	Fair/poor
Gender:*			
Male	418 (64.6)	189 (29.2)	40 (6.2)
Female	474 (61.4)	219 (28.4)	79 (10.2)
Education:*			
Less than high school	295 (51.0)	206 (35.6)	77 (13.4)
High school + some university	150 (64.1)	65 (27.8)	19 (8.1)
University graduates	437 (75.1)	126 (21.6)	19 (3.3)
Personal income:*			
Less than $30,000	528 (59.3)	276 (31.0)	86 (9.7)
$30,000 and over	145 (80.6)	27 (15.0)	—
Language proficiency:*			
English/French	710 (67.4)	280 (26.6)	64 (6.1)
No English/French	178 (49.6)	126 (35.1)	55 (15.3)
Years of stay in Canada:			
< 10 years	95 (68.8)	35 (25.4)	—
10+ years	601 (61.6)	284 (29.1)	91 (9.3)

Source: Computed from Canadian Community Health Survey, Cycle 3.1, Public Use Microdata File.

Note: Percentages in each cell show those who responded to that particular question; *** $p < 0.001$, ** $p < 0.01$, * $p < 0.05$; "—" denotes "cases less than 15, not appropriate to report."

TABLE 4: *Health Care Utilization and Health of Visible Minority Seniors by Language Proficiency and Years in Canada, 2005*

Indicators	Can converse in English/ French N (%)	Cannot converse in English/ French N (%)	p-value	Less than 10 years in Canada N (%)	10 years or more in Canada N (%)	p-value
Has chronic condition:						
yes	1,050 (89.1)	404 (91.8)	0.103	114 (74.5)	1,042 (91.0)	0.000
no	129 (10.9)	36 (8.2)		39 (25.5)	103 (9.0)	
Has regular medical doctor:						
yes	1,124 (95.3)	435 (98.9)	0.001	150 (98.0)	1,112 (97.0)	0.482
no	55 (4.7)	—		—	34 (3.0)	
Number of doctor's visits:						
1–6 times	762 (71.3)	248 (58.4)	0.000	112 (75.7)	691 (65.2)	0.000
7 times or more	306 (28.7)	177 (46.6)		36 (24.3)	369 (34.8)	
Consulted alternate health provider:						
yes	92 (7.8)	81 (18.5)	0.000	—	137 (12.0)	0.052
no	1,087 (92.2)	357 (81.5)		141 (93.4)	1,009 (88.0)	
Last time had flu shot:						
< 1 year	693 (85.2)	272 (96.8)	0.000	92 (90.2)	647 (86.8)	0.052
1 year or more	120 (14.7)	—		—	98 (13.2)	
Last time eyes examined:						
< 1 year	383 (70.7)	108 (56.5)	0.000	67 (67.7)	329 (63.5)	0.700
1–2 years	92 (17.0)	39 (20.4)		16 (16.2)	100 (19.3)	
2 years or more	67 (12.4)	44 (23.0)		16 (16.2)	89 (17.2)	
Last time visited dentist:						
< 1 year	334 (61.1)	84 (50.3)	0.045	48 (57.1)	295 (58.8)	0.017
1–2 years	91 (16.6)	37 (22.2)		—	104 (20.7)	
2 years or more	122 (22.3)	46 (27.5)		27 (32.1)	103 (20.5)	

Source: Computed from the Canadian Community Health Survey, Cycle 3.1, Public Use Microdata File.

Note: Percentages in each cell show those who responded to that particular question; "—" denotes "cases smaller than 15, not appropriate to report."

THIRTEEN

ABORIGINAL HEALING

David Young PhD

INTRODUCTION

Aboriginal healing is a holistic approach that addresses imbalances in the interaction of mind, body, emotions, and spirit. Aboriginal healers, who often refer to themselves as "medicine people," usually acquire their expertise through apprenticeship with elders who are willing to pass on their knowledge to those who have the qualities necessary to safeguard the sacred traditions and use them for the benefit of others. However the necessary knowledge is acquired, the process is lengthy as it involves learning about complex matters such as how and when to harvest and combine herbal medicines and animal parts, how to conduct sacred ceremonies, how to address the psychological and spiritual needs of those who come for help, and how to serve as an intermediary between the spirit and human worlds. An effective healer combines several roles, such as herbalist, physician, psychological counsellor, and priest. He or she is also frequently involved in a leadership role in the community, which requires political astuteness. Although healers have some knowledge of all of these different factors, they often specialize in one aspect, such as herbal knowledge or ceremonies.

Working with Aboriginal healers, especially if one is not a member of the Aboriginal community, is also a complex process with many pitfalls. In this chapter, the author, an anthropologist, discusses some of the theoretical issues and methods he employed in researching Aboriginal healing over a number of years. While some of these issues and methods have long been central to field-oriented research disciplines, others are controversial, especially to investigators who entertain the notion that to do science, one must remain as objective as possible.

PARTICIPANT OBSERVATION
Theoretical Considerations
The basic method of a field-oriented research discipline is participant observation, which involves living with a group of people and participating in their daily lives until what one sees and hears begins to make sense. The first step is to look and listen with as few preconceptions as possible. Over time, certain behavioural and linguistic themes are repeated often enough that they appear to have significance for the people involved. At this point, it is possible to begin asking meaningful questions about these themes.

As one's informants explain what they are doing and saying, it is important that the anthropologist take them seriously. This involves more than simply writing down what one is seeing and hearing. It involves attempting to constrain a sense of skepticism about explanations that are at odds with one's own beliefs about the nature of reality. As noted anthropologist Gregory Bateson (Bateson and Bateson, 1987) put it, the investigator should attempt to suspend disbelief in what he or she is being told and "act as if" he or she believes it. This does not mean that researchers have to give up their own belief systems, since that is impossible. It means that they must be open to what they are hearing and seeing for the purpose of experiencing what reality would look like, at least temporarily, if one were to adopt the basic assumptions, beliefs, and values of one's informants. This type of "acting as if" one believes might seem dishonest to some, but it is an important first step in learning to empathize with another culture.

The goal of participant observation is to develop an "emic" or inside perspective on the culture one is studying. This does not mean that it is possible for an outsider to become a "native," but it does mean that an outsider can learn enough about a culture to understand what is happening around him or her and to respond appropriately. This process of becoming "enculturated" is a little bit like learning a language in that a culture is similar to a grammar. In most situations there are a number of possibilities in terms of appropriate responses. How these behavioural options are linked together to form a behavioural strategy is dictated by cultural rules. It is possible to learn a good deal about cultural grammars, even though one may never be aware of all of the subtleties apparent to someone who was born and raised in that society.

Examples

Although I have worked with several different Aboriginal healers, the medicine person with whom I have had the greatest contact is Russell Willier, a northern Cree healer from the Sucker Creek Reserve in Alberta.

I discovered by accident that Russell Willier is a healer. In 1984, I was associated with an interdisciplinary team involving the University of Alberta and the Provincial Museum of Alberta (now the Royal Alberta Museum) to document the traditional skin-tanning procedures of Russell and his wife Yvonne. After a foundation of trust was established, Russell revealed that he is a healer, having received his medicine bundle, via his father and grandfather, from his great-grandfather, Moostoos, one of the most respected medicine men of his day.

When the skin-tanning project was completed, a revised interdisciplinary team initiated the Psoriasis Research Project, whose mandate was to document Russell Willier's treatment of several non-Native individuals afflicted with psoriasis, an itchy, scaly disease that is notably difficult to treat. We settled upon psoriasis since changes in the condition are so easy to observe. Russell was eager to participate in the project since he wished the efficacy of Aboriginal healing to be recorded in "black and white" for everyone to see. This decision was controversial at the time. Today, however, there are numerous medicine people who recognize the need to document medicine beliefs and practices before the old-time practitioners die. Over the following five years, I and other members of the research team visited the Sucker Creek Reserve frequently, staying overnight or longer, to interview Russell and to participate in healing rituals such as sweat lodge ceremonies. The results of this experience appear in the book *Cry of the Eagle: Encounters with a Cree Healer* (Young, Ingram, & Swartz, 1989).

Early in the fieldwork, I was exposed to stories, particularly about spirits, that seriously challenged my own beliefs about the nature of reality. For example, Russell revealed that Moostoos was one of the few medicine people of his day who could kill a *wittigo*, an evil creature created by a bad medicine man from ice, straw, and dirt. On one occasion, several medicine people succeeded in capturing a *wittigo* that was bothering their area but were unable to kill it. After having melted icicles coughed up by the *wittigo*, thereby destroying its power, Moostoos was able to kill the *wittigo* with an axe.

Moostoos was most famous for conducting shaking tipi ceremonies, attended by large numbers of people. The procedure was to mark off a circular area on the ground and to cover this area with sharpened skewers driven into the ground. A tipi was then constructed over the skewers, after which Moostoos would be securely bound hand and foot, wrapped in a blanket and tied again with leather thongs. He was then placed outside the entrance to the tipi. When the witnesses present began to chant and pray, Moostoos would suddenly fly through the entrance, the tipi would begin to shake, and spirits would begin speaking from different locations in the air around the tipi. Eventually the blanket and thongs would fly out of the entrance and Moostoos would emerge, unbound and unhurt.

I was apparently successful in being able to "act as if" I believed such stories, with the result that I and my family were invited to a rattle ceremony, a modern-day version of the shaking tipi ceremony, conducted by a healer on a reserve in 1987. The ceremony was held inside a log building with males seated on one side and females on the other. The altar was set up in the middle, where the healer was bound. Before beginning the ceremony, the healer cautioned that anyone who was skeptical should leave. Otherwise, he would suddenly find himself outside in the snow after the ceremony began. By this time, I had witnessed enough unusual events in the course of my fieldwork that I was able to go further than merely "suspending disbelief" and take the rattle ceremony quite seriously.

After the healer was bound, the lights were turned off, luminescent rattles began to fly around the tightly packed room (one of which bumped me on the head), and a variety of spirits entered to answer questions and conduct healing. At the conclusion of the ceremony, the lights were turned on and the healer was found at the back of the room, unbound and apparently in a daze. In the ensuing silence, food was shared and people began to file out quietly to return home.

I did not know how to offer an explanation to myself or others of the events I had witnessed in the rattle ceremony, but I felt very fortunate to have been invited to one of the most sacred ceremonies of Canadian Aboriginal people. My attitude at the time was that it was premature to attempt an explanation. I did not seriously begin to grapple with the issue of how to explain such experiences until 1994, when I and a colleague, Jean-Guy Goulet, edited a book on how anthropologists deal with experiences in other cultures that change their lives (Young & Goulet, 1994).

This attitude of suspending disbelief and taking what I witnessed and heard seriously, without attempting to devise explanatory models, was maintained throughout my fieldwork with Russell Willier. The Psoriasis Research Project, conducted partly in an inner-city health clinic in Edmonton, demonstrated that Aboriginal healing ceremonies were able to help non-Native patients afflicted with psoriasis, even though they had received little help from conventional Western medicine. After the project was formally concluded, two young people, one from Edmonton and one from Ontario, were treated for psoriasis on the Sucker Creek Reserve, with spectacular results (Young, Morse, Swartz, & Ingram, 1988). Both patients were photographed on four different occasions: immediately before the healing ceremonies, immediately after the healing ceremonies, three months later, and nine months after the ceremonies had taken place. Both patients recovered from massive skin disruptions that had seriously interfered with their lives.

This photographic record has served to convince many non-Native people, including some professors and students in the medical school at the University of Alberta, that Aboriginal medicine should be taken more seriously than it has been in the past. As a sign of this change of attitude, the Department of Family Medicine at the University of Alberta has hired a full-time Aboriginal healer, Clifford Cardinal, on staff. Cardinal believes that part of his mandate is to educate non-Natives about Aboriginal beliefs and practices, and to document those beliefs and practices for posterity.

INTERPRETING ONE CULTURE TO ANOTHER
Meaningful Description
The goal of participatory observation is to describe a set of beliefs or practices in a way that translates the essential, rather than the literal, meaning. This is a type of hermeneutic exposition. To insist on literal accuracy is a form of scholarly fundamentalism that can seriously distort the reality that

is being described. A well-known example from Biblical scholarship is the saying of Jesus that it is easier for a camel to go through the eye of a needle than for a rich man to enter heaven. Taken literally, Jesus seems to be saying that it is impossible for a rich man to enter heaven. If a proper cultural context is supplied, however, one learns that the walled city of Jerusalem had several gates, one of which was called Eye of the Needle because the top of the gate was so low that a camel had to stoop to get through. Taken in its proper cultural context, Jesus was saying that it is difficult, rather than impossible, for a rich man to enter heaven.

Thus hermeneutic exposition involves presenting enough of the cultural context that the set of beliefs or practices being described appears to make sense to an outside audience. Cultural beliefs and practices are usually rational in the sense that they have a useful function within the context of the culture, even though they may make little or no sense if removed from their cultural setting.

Explanatory Models

Some researchers believe that the research task is finished when beliefs and practices have been described in such a way that they appear to be meaningful and reasonable to an outside audience. If this were the case, the role of research would be primarily educational, to promote understanding and tolerance of other societies. Other researchers, including myself, believe that scientific investigation does not have to stop with an adequate cultural description. It can go one step further and attempt to "explain" events that one has witnessed to an outside audience.

The type of explanation that will be satisfactory depends, of course, upon the nature of the audience. If the audience belongs to a culture that readily accepts supernatural events, a supernatural explanation of an unusual event may suffice. If members of the audience belong to a culture that considers "scientific" explanations the only satisfactory ones, however, the researcher can be faced with a major challenge. For example, if the researcher witnesses what Andrew Weil (2000) calls "spontaneous healing" of a patient being treated by an Aboriginal healer, explaining to a scientific audience that the apparently miraculous recovery was due to intervention by God or spirits would not be very helpful.

This does not mean, however, that the researcher is free to speculate about scientific explanations that might satisfy the outside audience but that would be completely alien to the culture of those being studied. In other words, the researcher is not free to provide an "etic" (outside) explanation that takes no account of the "emic" (inside) reality associated with an event that has been witnessed. His or her obligation is to explain the event in such a way that it makes sense to the scientific audience without doing violence to the cultural values, beliefs, and practices of those being studied.

One way to accomplish this sometimes difficult task is to use a "meta-model"—an explanation that is sufficiently broad to encompass both Indigenous and scientific explanations. There is no set procedure for developing a meta-model. A meta-model can require a considerable amount of creativity on the part of the researcher. This does not mean that constructing meta-models is an exercise in fantasy, totally devoid of scholarly merit. In fact, most useful models and theories are not derived systematically from empirical data but involve a leap of intuitive insight that is more akin to art than to science. A model or theory should be judged in terms of its heuristic value—that is, in terms of its usefulness in making sense of a body of empirical data. In brief, a meta-model incorporates both emic and etic elements.

Examples

In the course of conducting fieldwork with Russell Willier and other Aboriginal healers, I have taken part in numerous ceremonies, such as "sweats" and vision quests, in which I have seen and heard spirits while in an altered state of consciousness induced by the ceremony. Although I did not know how to explain such experiences, I was determined not to fall into the trap that has ensnared researchers who have dutifully written down what informants told them about spirits but who have been shocked when they encountered spirits themselves. Such encounters are rarely reported because they are not considered appropriate scientific data. This kind of attitude is patronizing in that it is based on the assumption that it is normal for members of traditional societies to see spirits and to entertain unscientific beliefs, but if the researcher does so, he or she must have some kind of problem.

In an article discussing my visionary experiences of spirits (Young, 1994), I entertained the following hypothesis:

> My initial reaction to these visions was that they represented intuitive, probably unconscious, insights of some sort. My "aesthetic"

hypothesis went something like this: To understand an unconscious insight, it must assume a form we can apprehend. The individual who has a vision somehow must externalize, energize, and anthropomorphize his/her insight. Such a phenomenon would not be a simple psychological projection in the way that projections are usually conceived. It would be a projection of energy which takes on an independent form for a limited period of time for the purpose of teaching or dialogue, after which it dissolves back into its source. Thus a "spirit" is akin to a work of art in that energy is molded into a concrete statement which takes on a life of its own in the sense that it has the capability of revealing something to its creator which is not always welcome but which cannot be ignored. (171–72)

I laid out the following criteria for developing a meta-model that does justice to the reality of one's experience without wreaking violence upon one's own world view or the world view of informants in the culture that provided the stimulus for the experience:

1. The model should be true to one's experience.
2. The model should not do violence to the views of one's informants.
3. The model should be broad enough to encompass the researcher's own interpretation, as well as the interpretations of his or her informants.
4. The model should be capable of communicating meaning to individuals in the researcher's own culture.

The attempt to construct a meta-model involves what Bandler and Grinder (1982) have called "reframing"—trying out different explanations until one is found that serves the purpose. A meta-model is a type of myth that provides a bridge between experience and explanation. It is a myth in the sense that it is a metaphorical device that should not be taken in a highly literal way. This does not mean that it is untrue. In fact, all models are probably metaphorical in the sense that they attempt to depict complex relationships in a simplified form.

In attempting to understand spirits, it is not necessary to assume that they have an ontological existence independent of one's mind. Instead, spirits may be comprised of material from unconscious levels of the mind that break through into consciousness under the right conditions. If this unconscious material can be provided with a recognizable form, then it can serve as an internal hermeneutic bridge between the unconscious and conscious levels of the mind, thereby providing access to deep intuitive insights that are otherwise inaccessible.

Providing unconscious material with a recognizable form is a creative task akin to the production of a work of art in which the creator utilizes psychic energy to create a form that takes on a life of its own for a time. These forms that appear in dreams or visions are not hallucinations but messengers from a level of the mind in which the individual is connected with what Tillich (1951) called the Ground of our Being or what Buddhists call the Buddha Nature that underlies all of reality. Aboriginal people in Canada call these messengers the Grandfathers and Grandmothers (Young, Pompana, Spitzer, & Candler, 1996). One sophisticated Aboriginal healer told me that the Grandfathers and Grandmothers are like Carl Jung's concept of archetypes that dwell in the most primitive parts of the brain. Although these messengers from the "Unconscious" are given form by the individual who encounters them, they are at least partially autonomous in the sense that they are not merely projections of unconscious desires and fears. They bring information and insights from a realm in which everything is connected. Thus they transcend individual experience.

The role of ceremony and ritual in traditional cultures is to create an atmosphere in which participants are encouraged to enter an altered state of consciousness in which normal preconceptions and perceptions are temporarily set aside so that visions can occur. As Russell Willier conceded to me on one occasion, the healer sets the stage for spirits to appear. For example, in a "sweat," the intense heat forces one to focus upon controlling skin temperature; the rhythmic chanting and beating of the drum has a hypnotic influence; and the words of the healer encourage participants, who are in a highly suggestible state, to open themselves to the healing power and insights provided by messenger spirits. In my article on meta-models, I argue that:

> Regardless of the level from which it [unconscious material] comes, however, it has an urge to make itself known. If the urge is powerful enough, it will evade all of the normal psychological and cultural barriers and take on a form which is so realistic and compelling that it cannot be ignored. To insist on calling such visions hallucinations is a blatant expression of positivistic thinking. It could be argued

that the deeper levels of our being have at least as much reality as the role-playing that we normally associate with everyday life. If this is so, the forms that appear in visions should not be ignored, but treated with respect. (Young, 1994, p. 187)

In brief, according to the meta-model proposed above, a spirit is the product of a creative act in which energy and insight from the deepest levels of what Jung called the collective unconscious are given recognizable form in dreams and visions by an individual in the right state of mind. This state of mind can happen naturally, as in night dreaming, or it can be induced by ceremonies designed to relax normal modes of perception and conception. Thus spirits should not be regarded as hallucinations but as messengers from deeper levels of experience that come with the power to heal and with insights that can change one's life. They are thus to be welcomed.

TAKING META-MODELS BACK TO ONE'S INFORMANTS

If a meta-model makes sense to an outside audience, it can be deemed to be at least partially valid, in terms of successfully crossing the cultural boundary. Its validity in terms of preserving the emic meaning system it attempts to explain, however, can only be established by taking the meta-model back to one's informants and seeing if it makes sense to them. When I took the above meta-model back to my informants, the response was usually something like this, "Well, your explanation seems to be un-necessarily abstract, but it makes sense to me. It fits with what I have told you about the Grandfathers and Grandmothers."

If a meta-model passes this double-edged validity test, it can serve as a useful device for cross-cultural communication. It can also provide a use-ful contribution to our understanding of phenomena such as spontaneous healing. This does not mean, of course, that a valid meta-model is neces-sarily true in some ultimate sense. There might be other meta-models that might work just as well. Also, a meta-model that works well at one time and place might fail miserably under other circumstances. Thus meta-models must be open-ended and sufficiently flexible to be revised as needed. They are metaphors that must be judged in terms of their heuristic value.

SPONTANEOUS HEALING

Spontaneous healing is frequently observed when conducting research with Aboriginal medicine people. It is not uncommon to see individuals who have not received much help from Western medicine be "cured" in an Aboriginal ceremony. Understanding such events within the context of Western science is not easy. The most common explanation is that illnesses subject to spontaneous healing are most likely to be psychosomatic, in that emotional or mental conditions, usually stress-related, play a large role in somatic expression. A highly meaningful event in which faith on the part of the patient is reinforced is sometimes sufficient to trigger a dramatic healing event.

Such an explanation differs sharply from that of an Aboriginal healer, who is likely to attribute the recovery to the Great Spirit, working through spirit intermediaries assisted by the healer. The first explanation appears to be scientific, whereas the second explanation appears to be religious. The seemingly wide gulf between these explanations, however, can be lessened or overcome with the type of meta-model described above.

Aboriginal healers usually are quick to acknowledge that psychological factors, including faith, play an important role in healing. Other factors, such as herbal remedies, also may be involved. Aboriginal healers emphasize, however, that one should not forget that healing is assisted by power that transcends individual patients and healers. The role of a skilled healer is to bring all of these different factors together in a sacred ceremony that creates an atmosphere conducive to the activation of healing powers that lie both within and beyond the individual. Thus a healing ceremony is holistic in that it addresses biological, mental, and spiritual conditions and needs.

The ultimate source of the power that is tapped in a healing ceremony can be debated. Is it psychic energy that is always available to the individual, but that is rarely used? Or is it energy that transcends the individual— energy that comes from the Creator? It is not particularly fruitful to try to determine which of these hypotheses has greater merit. The meta-model described above encompasses both explanations with its argument that, under certain circumstances, it is possible to open oneself to power and insight from deeper, unconscious levels of the mind. Although such power and insight are psychological, they are at a level of the mind where the individual psyche is in touch with everything else in the universe. In other words, such power and insight are not confined to individual resources.

This is a level in which science and religion come together. This is a level that invites Aboriginal healers and scholars from the biological sciences, social sciences, and humanities to investigate phenomena such as spontaneous healing. The meta-model that may evolve as a result of such interdisciplinary investigation will be much richer and more comprehensive than the rudimentary beginnings described in this chapter.

CONCLUSION

Aboriginal healing is a complex, holistic endeavour that is worthy of serious study by Western researchers. It is worthy of study because, although rooted in ancient traditions, Aboriginal healing is very modern in its emphasis upon the interaction of mind, body, and spirit. This is a theme that appears with increasing frequency in Western literature as researchers learn more about the complex factors that influence health and disease.

Working with Aboriginal healers is not easy since it requires a degree of commitment to experiencing a different culture that places the researcher outside the confines of "normal science." It also challenges one's conceptions of reality and may effect significant change in one's values and even in one's personality. Working with Aboriginal healers is difficult for another reason as well. There is a certain amount of suspicion of outsiders who attempt to participate in Aboriginal communities and cultures. There is, of course, good reason for this as Aboriginal people have been severely exploited and continue to suffer various degrees of discrimination from the larger society. A common response from members of Aboriginal communities is, "You have taken our lands and traditional ways of doing things. Now you want to exploit our sacred knowledge as well."

One of the greatest challenges facing researchers who wish to document Aboriginal healing practices and come to a better understanding of their efficacy, is learning how to work with Aboriginal healers in a way that safeguards traditional knowledge from exploitation by those who might wish to utilize it for commercial gain. This will require collaborative effort by Aboriginal healers and Western researchers. This collaborative path is fraught with potential difficulties and misunderstandings, but the rewards are well worth the effort: satisfaction on the part of Aboriginal people that their traditional knowledge is finally being recognized as a form of "indigenous science" and a greater understanding on the part of Western researchers concerning the holistic nature of health and healing.

REFERENCES

Bandler, R., & Grinder, J. (1982). *Reframing: Neuro-linguistic programming and the transformation of meaning.* Moab, UT: Real People Press.

Bateson, G., & Bateson, M.C. (1987). *Angels fear: Towards an epistemology of the sacred*. New York: Macmillan.

Tillich, P. (1959). *Theology of Culture*. New York: Oxford University Press.

Weil, A. (2000). *Spontaneous healing: How to discover and enhance your body's natural ability to maintain and heal itself*. New York: Random House.

Young, D. (1994). Visitors in the night: A creative energy model of spontaneous visions. In D.E. Young & J.-G. Goulet (Eds.), *Being changed by cross-cultural encounters: The anthropology of extraordinary experience* (pp. 166–96). Peterborough, ON: Broadview.

Young, D.E., & Goulet, J.-G. (Eds.). (1994). *Being changed by cross-cultural encounters: The anthropology of extraordinary experience*. Peterborough, ON: Broadview.

Young, D., Ingram, G., & Swartz, L. (1989). *Cry of the eagle: Encounters with a Cree healer*. Toronto: University of Toronto Press.

Young, D., Morse, J., Swartz, L., & Ingram, G. (1988). The psoriasis research project: An overview. In David E. Young (Ed.), *Health care issues in the Canadian north* (pp. 76–88). Edmonton: Boreal Institute for Northern Studies.

Young, D., Pompana, C., Spitzer, D., & Candler, C. (1996). A hermeneutic exposition of a plains healer's concept of "the Grandfathers." *Anthropos, 92*, 115–28.

FOURTEEN

REFLECTIONS OF A CREE HEALER'S PARTNER

Delores Cardinal

VERY LITTLE CAN BE FOUND in the literature on the kind of partnership a Cree healer has with his wife in providing care for the community. Delores Cardinal agreed to provide us with some background so that we understand the complexity of Indigenous ways of healing. The editors of this volume provided her with questions in several areas of the healing tradition, which she reflected upon; she then worked with us in interviews to address them, as well as to add other perspectives. The following represents selected remarks that she and her husband, Clifford, made.

CLIFFORD'S DESCRIPTION OF ABORIGINAL HEALING TRADITION

"Medewin" Healing Society

Delores participates in a select group of people who are gifted in healing. This group is distinctive because they have given themselves to the Indigenous way of healing—that is, they represent a healing tradition within Indigenous societies. Their healing abilities are passed on to those they trust; this means that the knowledge stays within a very limited and responsible healer "specialization." It includes people like the following: Gilbert Cardinal, the late Peter Shirt, Robert Smallboy, Raymond Harris, Frank Foolscrow, Morris Lewis, Jim Canopotato, Jimmie Driever, Machees Red Crow, Sam McGilvary, Peter Cardinal Clark and Lloyd Cardinal, Mugalair Cardinal, and my kokum, Louise Witford. We are going to be talking about traditional knowledge and how medicine was practised by my family. My own connection to this group began very early...when I was five. I received visions about healing, and these were followed by teachings from matriarch Rosie Bruno Cardinal from Wolf Lake, Alberta, and then by prophecies as told by the late Jim Banks, who was a half-brother to Big Bear through their common dad through Black Powder. This background and history has been documented by a number of old people, including Stand Cuthand and most recently by sundance leader and Poundmaker's Lodge, Jerome Tootoosis. We talked about my *mosum*, my *mosum* in the third person, and how he escaped the battles of 1885 between the Cree people and General Middleton from the Canadian Army or the North West Mounted Police. This group has a long and deep history in this part of the world.

Elements of Healing Tradition

We should begin by acknowledging that this healing tradition has a history too, that is, that there is an important tribal component to it: the Woodland Cree, the Plains people, Saulteaux, and Stoney people all had an impact on the way healing was conducted. In fact, the Stoney people had an impact on the way ceremonies were conducted right up to 1975, with the coming of the Arapaho teachings through the late Raymond Harris. It is important to know that, during that period, ceremony was not part of everyday life. In fact it was hidden. It was not something that took place every day in Indigenous community life. In fact it is (and was) a hidden aspect. All the ceremonies of Saddle Lake, Goodfish Lake, and Kehewin, most of them were conducted at night; that is, they are not open for everyone to see and participate in. So, for example, the old men might make a sweat way out in the wilderness, where certain old men would converge to do the ceremonies. This tradition continued until 1972, when it was openly practised by my family, when I turned 17, also at Woods Point where I was initiated into this healing society.

Crucial Role of Women in Traditional Healing

Most importantly, what we want to speak about is the role that women have and still continue to play. In ceremonies, it was a long-forgotten responsibility, but one which my mother Rose held. She was always the focal point in all the ceremonies. This means that she organized the vision quests, she organized the *witokowin* (great community feasts), which were held at my home at which I was already at an early age a young "priest." I did what my mother told me to do, and my role was simply to follow the instructions and do the ceremonies that my mother organized. When she died, that responsibility fell to my partner, Delores. All aspects of these ceremonies for healing, the sundance, fastings, night lodges, all of the logistics, all aspects of the ceremonies, organization of the elements of the ceremonies, all this was the responsibility of the women.

The belief that it is the man doing the healing alone has always fallen below the proper standards, even with the personnel who were thoroughly gifted by the Great Spirit. It was thought that a healer was given certain rights and certain limitations; the woman had a role within that responsibility... in that wheel of responsibility. As with everything else, along with birthing and giving birth to the ensuing generations, the amount of responsibility is great within women's lives. How can this be measured out or studied separately at this point remains to be seen. I think this exercise will prove that there is a hidden agenda for us from the Great Spirit; however, there hasn't been a time when men around the campfire or men around the tipi have ever discussed the role that their women had regarding each ceremony. For example, I heard a story where this well-known healer was denouncing the fact that he had given his wife a certain amount of power. He expressed regrets during a period of time when they were not getting along and he apparently took that power to do the healing back from his wife. The reason why we undertook this task (to speak about the healing traditions) was knowing that 80% of our healing knowledge is gone, and those who know are dying or already dead. There is no other way to protect it or to save this knowledge. Some of my people have been saying, well, someone in the future is going to get it (back) through a very gifted young person, who will receive the knowledge. I don't see all the knowledge as being dispensable this way; because the knowledge is too diverse, it is too specific in nature for each healer. One factor is that each of us has our own specialty, and all of us have our own role in communal ceremonies, like the pipe ceremonies, and sweat and sundance ceremonies. And who needs each of these specialties is not determined by the community, but by the person having received a gift. The role of women, well, one cannot say it is pivotal to its own survival, but it has always been part of the whole circle, the great mystery as well as one of the most secretive ceremonies, the full moon ceremonies, that are now practised by just about every tribal community in Canada and the U.S. These ceremonies were always there before the coming of the Europeans. The full moon ceremony also served as a calendar, a way of preparing the community and the camp as they moved from one place to another. And even all that responsibility has been noted by scholars.

All healers have knowledge not determined by the community but received as individuals from the spirit world. The knowledge of women is not separate from that...their knowledge has always been part of the great circle of knowledge, and they always were part of the four great ceremonies we practised in the community (sweats, vision quest, thirst dance, shaking tent) before White people came.

Then there is the fact that it was the women who did all the preparing of the camp in the community. Women owned the homes and organized the camp's supplies. They were in charge of the food supplies. Even Mandelbaum said that roles were determined by survival, and by the chief. But we must bear in mind who has insights into the camp's supplies. Who does the chief listen to at night? Who does he talk to every night when he has to decide where to go and what to do?

All those things that healers are unwilling to surrender, that is, (to give) a certain amount of their power to their partners, the decision now to document the knowledge will make it available. That decision was well received by Gordon Steinhauer, Albert Desjarlais, Ron Kristman, Keith Varslikan, and at least six other healers from Canada and the U.S. That role was given to me. At a certain point it just so happened that the University of Alberta approached me, and when that happened, because it was planned way before now, the people felt that the Creator had answered our prayers. But the defining elements and the other healing ceremonies have been documented so well by different authors, in both Canada and the U.S....for example, the sweat has been well documented, the sundance, the shaking tent, have been documented and how they are practised...and all the dimensions of each lodge has been documented. What hasn't been documented is the power and responsibility that the Creator gave to women. So we start now by discussing the hows and whys of the roles that women have and had. How it affected each healing practice, as each person comes in to ask for help, at which part does the woman's job begin? As I mentioned earlier, my own mother arranged all of this for me before I was old enough to even plan anything...even plan my own life. The sweat lodges, the vision lodges, the night lodges, all of those were organized by my parents but primarily by my mother. How she got knowledge, all I know is she was raised by traditional people, by ceremonial people, the same way that my own partner was raised. I think by having her explain the roles she has played throughout each ceremony, and even co-ordinating hundreds of people at a given time, I think this will explain some of the intricate and diverse responsibilities even in doing a simple ceremony.

DELORES'S REFLECTIONS ON PARTNER'S ROLE IN CREE HEALING

First of all, I am grateful for the opportunity to speak of my role and my responsibilities as a medicine man's wife. This is a role I have taken upon myself in living with a medicine man. My story begins a very long time ago, in my early life. I was raised in a traditional family, and we practised traditional ceremonies and ways of life. So whatever I have it has been passed on to me from those who have gone before, from my teachers. I was raised to be humble, to respect the elders of our people, to care for the old folk.

I did not know my great grandparents, since they both died in 1956 and I was born in 1957. Even though I never knew them, I was told stories about great grandmother, how she was such a fine lady. She was also a healer. Sometimes old medicine men passed their knowledge on to daughters. Maybe that was how she was such a good woman. In addition, very early I learned from my grandmother about medicine plants, because she had knowledge about plants that heal. With her I just picked medicines, although I did hear stories from the medicine people who came to her for the medicines she had collected.

Everything was done at night, and I wondered why. Perhaps it was at night because our people were colonized and they had to do the ceremonies at night so that their knowledge could be kept and passed on to the younger generations. I guess that's why everything was done at night. That's how I remember how my early life was like.

After I began going with Clifford, I had to learn from his mother. I had to learn a great deal, many ceremonies, many things like the sweat lodge, the night lodge, and other ceremonies. Frankly, I don't know why the partners of medicine men have not written about their lives—this is important work.

Maybe it is because they didn't want other people to know about it for fear of the repercussions. Maybe because it is difficult learning all you have to learn. I learned most of what I know from my mother-in-law. She was a very kind lady, and she cared for everyone in the most graceful way. If I made a mistake, she corrected me in a gentle way; I never knew her to be mean about anything. In fact, once Clifford and I were married, she became my best friend. When I was pregnant with my son, she was right beside me. In all the years that Clifford and I have been married, I never had a difference with her on anything. We did everything together—dried meat, stored food for winter, cooked. She told me many stories and that one way I learned so many things. I loved and cared for her until the very end of her life. She told me that she would be with us on life's path, and she would even be with us after she walked into the next life.

Then, about 15 years ago, my grandpa gave me my great grandmother's medicine bundle. But I do not know the medicines in that bundle, since it has to be transferred to me. I asked when I will know the medicines of the bundle. I was told that the knowledge, it will come in dreams. I've not had those dreams yet. But it is a very old bundle, long before Whites came to this country. I take very good care of that bundle and value it a great deal.

As Clifford matured as a medicine man, I had to learn many of the ceremonies. I had to pay special attention to these ceremonies, because they were different, depending upon the illness. It could be a real challenge. I guess one thing I had to learn to face was my fear...that the people we were working with would not survive. I had to totally have faith that a person would be helped with the knowledge that our ancestors left behind for us.

Then, I've had to learn where and how to pick some medicines. Clifford has taken me to many, many places for medicines. The most recent thing I've done is climb a mountain and pray nearby with our sacred pipes. I always have to prepare myself and make sure there are properly prepared medicines for our people. I have to make sure that they are picked at just the right moment. Most of our picking takes place from spring to early fall, but they are picked all over the place. After picking them, it is my responsibility to see that they are properly handled, that none of them are touched by anyone else but Clifford and me. Then I have to make sure that we have enough medicines for a whole year of healing, since we can only get them at a certain season. We now find that we have to go farther and farther to find medicines, away from pollution and the development that is going on in the province. We have to travel so far to get clean medicines.

Then we have to pay attention to stories on how to pick medicines. For example, my mother-in-law told me how to pick the bark from a certain tree, not just any of the bark anywhere, but the bark at a particular spot, from a particular side of the tree. Our medicines can be very complicated now.

All our healing protocols are based on prayer. That is, prayer is offered through the pipes, and to the grandfathers, both of which are concerned with our well-being. They are around us all the time. They have encouraged us to keep our ceremonies just as they were always done; we want to keep the most ancient of our ways.

BACKGROUND ON HEALING TRADITION

There are many stories about how we understand sickness. We have a word for what we do: it is the Cree word *ownatawihiwew*, which says that we provide healing medicine for people. There are others who are gifted for helping people in Cree culture, but that word describes what we are.

We know there are sicknesses now that we did not have before contact with White society, so there were pre-contact medicines, and then there are post-contact medicines. At the point where Whites began to come, there were new sicknesses that we had never seen before, so the medicine people did not know how to deal with them. We lost a lot of people at that time, including medicine people. I don't know why so many old people are now blind among our people. Why is this? After contact, we had to learn how to cope with so many new sicknesses. We are still learning about new illness today.

Basically today, we see illness coming from four different sources. We can group them together under the following words: germs, environment, lifestyle, and spiritual.

First of all, we work with people who have a germ of some sort. We have worked with individuals who have hepatitis, TB, whooping cough, influenza, and HIV, to name a few. We know that we have to provide medicine that will allow people to get rid of these germs.

Then there are those who are reacting to the environment in some way. Today we have to treat people with respiratory ailments, allergies, and asthma, and all of these are from the environment we live in. We also see reactions to pollution, such as different types of cancers, moulds, wood-burning reactions, sores, and rashes. We also have patients who have difficulties with altitude or have brain dysfunctions. Some of them have environmental illnesses dealing with water: beaver fever, colon cancer, bowel syndromes, etc.

Next, there are those illnesses that derive from a poor lifestyle: poor hygiene, overcrowded homes, poor nutrition, and unclean living places. We see patients who overuse narcotics, who use street drugs, and of course those who are alcoholic. Besides these, there are illnesses that relate directly to lifestyle, like promiscuity, prostitution, unsettled domestic life, etc. Some of our patients are suicidal, and this is very difficult. Some of them are totally welfare dependent, which destroys their sense of personal worth; some are illiterate; some are school dropouts without much hope of getting ahead; and some are in dire straits because there is very poor health promotion in their communities. Many of our communities suffer from various kinds of abuse: physical, mental, emotional, spiritual. The colonialization of our people has brought about great problems. Now we see loss of language, loss of self-esteem, and terrible forms of peer pressure. We see many people who have had cultural loss; they do not know the ceremonies, they do not know their history, and they see their friends dying younger and younger without much hope. There is a high morbidity rate among our people. Even ceremonies have changed, with some handing out handfuls of brown sugar as some kind of medicine. This has a very negative impact on people's sense of who they are, as well as on their physical well-being.

Finally, there are illnesses coming from spiritual decline. We see people who have strong envy of what others have, and they carry out vendettas against them. There are curses that are laid against people, which makes people subject to bad luck, such as inability to hunt, trap, or fish for themselves. In addition, spiritual decline means an increase in psychoses, with paranoia and schizophrenia. We have patients with obsessions, who just don't know how to deal with a life that doesn't seem to have any borders or boundaries. Some of them experience a reversal of roles, so that some of them can't judge right from wrong anymore. We have found that we can have a good impact on spiritual illnesses, if we can get to them immediately. But still, there are many we find it very difficult to treat because they have complications from other illnesses. This, combined with spiritual decline, makes the case very trying.

CREE PARTNER ROLES AND RESPONSIBILITIES

We receive patients from all over the country and I never know when I get up what we will have to deal with during the day. I don't know who will call or what illness we will be facing. I have to be prepared mentally for the different eventualities. I must make all the arrangements for these people.

I have never bothered to take notice of how much time I take to make arrangements for Clifford's patients. Every patient that calls or shows up at our home is likely to be different. We have been following the same protocol for many years. Many of the people that come are familiar with how Clifford does this doctoring, so I really don't have to prepare them very much. But I always tell the people before they arrive to make sure that they are in no rush at all. If they tell me they are rushing, I advise them to choose a time when they don't have to be in such a rush. Most of our healing is done in the evening.

What we do first is that people present a traditional offering to Clifford in recognition of his knowledge. They come with tobacco as a gift for him to listen to them and try to help them. Then we ask the people when they started to get ill. I make tea and we sit and listen to them. Then Clifford will tell me what ceremony he will perform and then I have to prepare things for the ceremony. If it is some kind of medicine that is mixed I might have to do that. Then I assist in the ceremony, depending on what it is for. I do this day and night. This is the job I have had for over 30 years as a healer's partner.

I try very hard to treat everyone the same. I try to make them feel comfortable. I try to make a cozy feeling in my home, so they will feel safe and secure. I try to show them that my door is open to them whenever they need help. Along with my children, we have tried to keep our home calm and peaceful so that people feel good about being there, and the ceremony is carried out in a quiet environment.

It is also my responsibility to remember the person and the treatment, so we keep small records, mostly so I can remember all we treat. We keep documents on each patient but we keep all this very confidential. We do not share our knowledge with anyone. Everyone can come in complete confidence that the problem will be between us and the patient.

At the end of the ceremonies, we provide some food for our patients. Sometimes I have to cook early in the morning if we know how many people are coming. We can have as many as 50 patients in a week; sometimes when we go to the sundance, we will serve over 150 people in a 12-day period. It is very tiring, but we are happy that we can help so many people.

We use the pipe ceremony, the healing pipe ceremony. We also use the sacred smudge. This is passed down to us from generation to generation. We are the ones to be the role models to show our children how to do these things, so we can continue the teachings and the ceremonies that way we've been taught. Oftentimes now, we have these ceremonies in the late afternoon. However, some of them are held at night. The youngsters do not understand why we would hold a ceremony at night. They think maybe we are doing something hidden by this and are ashamed. The elders seem reluctant to tell them why it is held at night. This is not the way it is supposed to be. This is part of who we really are, and we should pass this knowledge on openly to them.

We believe healing is something that should be available for all people. It is important to be humble about the healing process, since we are only doing what so many of our ancestors have done, and we try very hard to help everyone. We even have White people who come for healing, and we treat all of them the same way.

COMMUNITY COMMITMENTS

It is obvious that our people are suffering. Many of them are quite sick, and many of them are dying prematurely. We are very concerned about this. We think we have to do something to put the community back on the right path. It is our responsibility now to try to teach about our ways so that youngsters will have some direction in life.

We try to have sweats and to bring both men and women into the sweat. We want them to be aware of the power of the pipes to help. We want to make them aware of the power in our ceremonies to help them.

Recently we have set up a moon-time ceremony for the young women. Many of them have great difficulty in adjusting to modern life, and many do not know the traditional teachings. Clifford suggested that I set up a moon-time ceremony at which I could teach the young women our protocols and help them adapt to the knowledge of who they are. Traditionally, women were recognized as having great power during their moon time, and they were careful not to disturb the ceremonies because of that. The point is that women expressed a different kind of power during their moon time.

Young women today think that this means there is something wrong with women. But this was not the case. Traditionally, it was not "bad power," it was just different power than what was available in the ceremonies. Our old people believed that there were several different kinds of power in the world; ceremonies had one, and women had another one. We have to teach women today because they are not raised to understand the traditional notions. For example, once a woman is no longer menstruating, she can sit in all the ceremonies without any difficulty. Even during our moon time it is merely having someone sit in for you so that there is no possibility of two different kinds of energy being present at the same time. Tradition just teaches us to take care to honour the ceremonies by assuring that the power of the ceremonies is absolute when they are being carried out. That way they can be the most effective to help people.

Throughout my career with Clifford, I just made sure that when ceremonies were being conducted, and it was during my moon time, that I was not close enough to have an influence on the spirits. When the ceremonies were finished, and the spirits had returned to the spirit world, I could come and go as was necessary—I could help with arrangements and all the other things that had to be done.

It is part of my role and responsibility now to teach people. I want to teach them the traditional ways, so that they will have something solid to hang on to. I have received teaching from great people, and I want to pass this on. That is another big the job that we have to do. That is why we want to work through the university so that this knowledge will be valued and passed on.

CONCLUSION

Earle H. Waugh

Olga Szafran

Rodney A. Crutcher

THROUGHOUT HISTORY, medical beliefs, treatments, and medical education have been rooted in the cultural traditions of societies. While the rise of scientific medicine in Western societies has altered or replaced many early beliefs and practices, cultural differences pertaining to health care and medicine persist. Nowhere is this more evident than in a country like Canada, where people from numerous ethnically diverse groups come in contact with Western medicine. Such diversity presents challenges for medical practitioners and medical educators.

At the Interface of Culture and Medicine has brought together a diverse collection of scholarly works on the topic of culture, health care, and medical education. The four parts of the book have drawn attention to the current Canadian issues at the interface of culture and medicine, these being end-of-life care, cultural competence and language, international medical graduates, and specific cultural groups (e.g., Aboriginals).

The chapters on culture and the end of life signal that the place of dying has undergone shifts, from home to hospital to home, while lifespan has been dramatically extended. Ethnicity and cultural differences are now important factors in end-of-life care. The works here have indicated trends that will require new forms of response. Aboriginal traditions are becoming even more important than was previously perceived, especially as Aboriginal demographics impact on health care. Current Canadian cultural and health institutions are challenged to optimally support service provision in a multicultural Canada. The Aboriginal community is only the most dominant of a number of groups that will change future patterns of care. Some shifts in priority must soon be made in researching the intersection of distinctive end-of-life views and the institutions that carry the burden of the dying. History will also continue to play a role in shaping future trends, whether from the collective memory of the Aboriginal community about past treatment, or from changes in our values from helping the elderly heal to living as effective a life as possible in the final stages of existence. On the basis of the chapters here, it is evident that professionals will encounter a clientele whose cultural assumptions differ significantly from those underpinning the training of many current health care providers. There will be significant systemic strain with a resultant call for greater training in health care provider cultural competence than has been the case until now.

It is evident that Canada's current shortage of physicians could be partly alleviated by the contributions of qualified, but currently unlicensed, international medical graduates (IMGs) residing in Canada. Many of these physicians are interested in re-entering health professional practice. The immigrant and refugee doctors in Canada have an untapped range of skills that may help relieve current shortages, while contributing to the provision of culturally competent care to our increasingly diverse population. The studies here have demonstrated that some progress is being made to integrate IMGs into the health professional workforce. Much remains to be done. Medicine's own culture may have to engage with IMGs in policy and professional standards discussions, so that more doctors can engage in some form of medical work while seeking both assessment and, in many cases, an upgrading of clinical skills. Culture has played a role in dampening skill usage, not necessarily because of medical standards, but from networks of control that may be more cultural than medical. A discussion of these issues among licensing bodies, IMG educators, professional associations, and heath authorities may be one catalyst for change. The chapters here provide support for a much greater engagement of the medical fraternity in policy change and argue for more research on the best way to bring about this modification for the benefit of all Canadians.

Language remains a key barrier to accessing health care across Canada, and language proficiency for health professional practice has been minimally researched. Culture's ties to language will not easily be swept aside by simply offering classes in English and French. With the influx of immigrants from the early 1990s to the foreseeable future, some sense of urgency attends the issue, and much work needs to be done in the area of culture and language in health care. While medicine struggles with the demands of multiple languages in service provision, more emphasis must be placed on strategies to assist with transitions for immigrant patients. Translations of standard medical terms, trained translators in urban areas dominated by certain language groups, and cadres of trained primary care professionals would go a long way to making health care more accessible. In an environment of cultural diversity, the cultural competence of health care professionals should facilitate the reduction of inequitable access in cross-cultural situations, the detection of culture-specific diseases, and the improvement of the health of culturally diverse populations.

Several chapters in this book make the case that Aboriginal systems of health need to be addressed in meaningful ways so that Canada's Aboriginal populations can at last participate openly and fully in the future of health care. For Canada to have a health care system that is inclusive, lacunae in medical education, medicine, government, and business need to be addressed. With a new generation of Aboriginal physicians challenging the system, research will be needed on how best to provide a bridge to these medical traditions.

Our collective work provides selected illustrative examples of areas where culture and medicine interface. The breadth of topics on culture and medicine are vastly greater than what is covered here. Additional areas where culture is also likely to have an important influence on medicine include geriatric care, the meaning of chronic diseases, sexual health and reproduction, child and adolescent health, and distinctive traditional/alternative medicines. These thematic areas should also be addressed in future research and writing.

We are acutely aware of the preliminary and cursory nature of our examination of issues at the interface of culture and medicine. Nevertheless, the chapters herein are offered as indicators of both work done and work to be done. We hope future studies will probe these and other issues with greater depth and increasing sophistication. This current collection is perhaps one of the starting points for such efforts.

CONTRIBUTORS

Heather Armson is an academic family physician working in the residency teaching unit at the University of Calgary. She has worked with international medical graduates for several years and was part of the development of a national Faculty Development Program for Teachers of International Medical Graduates.

John Baumber was with the Alberta International Medical Graduate Program since its inception in 2001 to 2008. He has extensive research and medical education experience and has held past leadership roles with the Medical Council of Canada. In 2008, Dr. Baumber was awarded the Order of the University of Calgary in recognition for his national and international contributions to medicine and medical education.

Margaret Brown is an Adjunct Research Fellow with the Hawke Research Institute, University of South Australia (SA) and a research consultant in advance care planning and advance directives. She is a social scientist who has researched ethical issues associated with dying and end-of-life decision-making and has published widely in this area. Margaret has been involved in numerous professional associations such as the Guardianship Board (SA), the Palliative Care Council (SA), and the Australian Bioethics Association. Her research in the community has contributed to changes in government policy and legislation. She has been the recipient of several major grants, including four Australian National Health and Medical Research Grants and other funded research projects.

Delores Cardinal is heir to a long tradition of plant/herbal healing called in Cree *ownatawihiwew*. This tradition drew upon the knowledge preserved in oral tradition and passed down from grandmother to daughter to granddaughter in an unbroken line for seven or more generations. Although schooled in Alberta schools, Delores received her career education at the feet of these great carriers of the *ownatawihiwew* tradition. Since her marriage to Clifford Cardinal, she has worked to provide healing for her people in tandem with him. As a member of a healing team, her collection and gathering processes are critical for the healing activity because the herbs and barks, etc. must be collected at just the right time, must be treated with the ultimate respect, and must be incorporated into a sacred rite that will provide the healing. Her skill is measured by the powerful way in which the rites provide benefit and the reputation of the healing tradition in the province and beyond.

Rodney A. Crutcher is an academic family physician and Professor in the Department of Family Medicine, University of Calgary. His activities in medical education include roles as a teacher, researcher, leader, and administrator across the medical education continuum. Dr. Crutcher is the University of Calgary's leader of the Sudanese Physician Reintegration Program, founding director of the Alberta International Medical Graduate Program (2000–2008), and a leader in international medical graduate initiatives in Canada.

Chantal Hansen is a Geographic Information Systems (GIS) analyst currently consulting for both the Faculty of Medicine and the Latin American Research Centre at the University of Calgary. A former geography teacher trained in Australia, she became interested in GIS as a teaching tool for her students. Chantal completed her MGIS degree in 2004. Her research interest is GIS for health and human services.

Marianna Hofmeister is the Alberta International Medical Graduate Program's Evaluation Coordinator. Her passion for the assessment and integration of international medical graduates into Canadian practice stems from a deep-seated commitment to social justice. Marianna has been in and around the Calgary health region as a laboratory technologist, patient, and researcher for more than 25 years.

Deidre Lake is the Director of Canadian Language Research and Consulting and the Co-creator and Program Manager for the Language Communication Assessment Project. She has been involved in a variety of research projects including the development of assessment tools for professional language proficiency.

Peggy Mann is a health human resources policy and program specialist. She has been involved with medical education and international medical graduates for a number of years, both from within the Ontario provincial government and as an independent consultant in Calgary.

Luz Palacios-Derflingher is a Research Associate in the Department of Medicine at the University of Calgary. Her areas of expertise are applied statistics, mixed effects models, and biostatistics. Luz holds a PHD in Statistics where she researched mixed effects models on unobservable response variables. She completed a post-doctoral fellowship in the Department of Family Medicine researching patient safety culture via the application of multilevel factor analysis.

Gayle E. Rutherford is an Assistant Professor in the Faculty of Nursing at the University of Calgary. She has a background in public health nursing practice, management, and education. She teaches in the areas of interprofessional education and community practice. Her research focuses on working with vulnerable populations in ways that help them to use their stories to work toward change. The writing of this book chapter arose from Gayle's previous work as a consultant when she was hired as a researcher on the project titled, "International Medical Graduates in Alberta: A Pilot Study of Professional and Personal Factors in Preparation for Practice."

Kamila Saieed graduated from University of Assiout, Egypt in 1987 and immigrated to Canada in 2001. Dr. Saieed made her journey to medicine in Canada through the Alberta International Medical Graduate Program and finished her family medicine residency program in 2006. In Egypt she worked as a family physician, and had postgraduate studies in pediatric psychiatry. Besides working with her patients, she enjoys reading, spending time with her family, and listening to music.

Sam Sheps is Professor in the School of Population and Public Health at University of British Columbia, Director of the Western Regional Training Centre for Health Services Research, and Program Director of the

MSC/PHD program. Dr. Sheps was a member of the British Columbia team of the Canadian Adverse Events Study. He was principal investigator on a Health Canada funded project assessing approaches to governance and safety in non-health industries, as well as a co-investigator on several projects applying his expertise in issues regarding patient safety derived from non-health, high reliability industry, specifically to emergency ward and intensive care units. Other research interests include surgical wait times, end-of-life, continuum of care issues, and primary care reform.

Denise L. Spitzer holds the Canada Research Chair in Gender, Migration and Health at the University of Ottawa where she is affiliated with the Institutes of Women's Studies and Population Health. Trained as a medical anthropologist, Dr. Spitzer is interested in the impact of marginalization on health and well-being and in the myriad ways in which people and communities resist marginalization. She works primarily with immigrant and refugee women and transnational migrant workers on a range of issues including: the intersections of work (both paid and unpaid), gender, and health; the impact of marginalization on the body; the relationship between policy and health; the influence of structural racism on the health and well-being of minority populations; and the salience of identity, social support, and social networks to health. In addition to graduate degrees in anthropology, Dr. Spitzer holds undergraduate degrees in biology and Chinese.

Juhee V. Suwal was a rural researcher in the Department of Family Medicine, University of Alberta (2005–2008). She received her PHD in sociology with specialization in demography from the University of Alberta in 2003. She was a lecturer on Padma Kanya Campus, Tribhuvan University, Nepal, teaching demography and statistics before coming to Canada in 1994. Currently, she is the Survey Unit Manager, Surveillance & Health Status Assessment Division, Alberta Health Services. She served as a member and executive member in a number of writers', women's, socio-cultural, and development-related non-profit organizations in Nepal, and in a number of academic associations in Canada. Her recent publications are in the areas of immigrant family caregivers in Canada and in maternal and infant mortality in Nepal. She has published short-story books in the Newar language of Nepal based on the socio-cultural situations of girls and women in Nepal. Her research interests include mortality, cause of death, health and mental health of vulnerable populations; and rural-urban comparison, ethnicity, and socio-cultural aspects in health and medicine.

Olga Szafran is the Associate Director (Research), Department of Family Medicine, University of Alberta. She obtained a Masters in Health Services Administration degree from the University of Alberta in 1985. Over the past 20 years, she has been involved in family practice research in the areas of prevention, physician practice patterns, medical education, international medical graduates, cultural competence, and health services research, and has published in these areas.

Roger Thomas is Professor of Family Medicine, University of Calgary. He taught sociology and anthropology at the University of Guelph. He obtained a medical degree from McMaster University, Canada. Over the years, he has held various positions including: Medical Superintendent at Bonavista Hospital, Newfoundland; Medical Superintendent at Mulanje Mission Hospital, Malawi; Associate Professor of Family Medicine East Carolina University and University of Toronto; Professor at University of Ottawa, Memorial University of Newfoundland, and the University of Calgary; and Cochrane Collaboration Coordinator, University of Calgary. Research interests include systematic reviews and meta-analyses; school, family and mentoring interventions to prevent children smoking; active learning; learning disabilities in children with neurological/behavioural problems; teaching medical students; effectiveness of influenza vaccine; screening for stomach cancer; home interventions for the elderly; palliative care; and telehealth.

Jean A.C. Triscott is Professor and Director of the Division for Care-of-the-Elderly, Department of Family Medicine, University of Alberta. She is also a consulting physician for the specialized geriatrics program, Capital Health, Edmonton, Alberta, and runs a Geriatric Assessment Clinic at the Glenrose Rehabilitation Hospital, Edmonton. As a physician, she has worked in geriatrics for 24 years. Her research interests are in health care in the elderly, impact of culture on health care, and dementia/end-of-life care.

Nigel Waters is a Distinguished Professor of Geography with more than 30 years of experience and research relating to Geographic Information Science. Currently, Dr. Waters is Director of the Center of Excellence for Geographic Information Science at George Mason University, Virginia, USA. Previously, he was Director of the Masters in Geographic Information Systems (MGIS) program at the University of Calgary. A former

President of the Western Canadian Association of Geographers and an Associate Editor of *GeoWorld*, Dr. Waters received his PHD from the University of Western Ontario.

David L.E. Watt is an Associate Professor and Graduate Coordinator in the Faculty of Education at the University of Calgary where he specializes in language assessment and language teaching. He has conducted research to establish rates of language acquisition for adult immigrants and is a co-creator of L-CAP program for the professional integration immigrant physicians in Alberta.

Earle H. Waugh is Professor Emeritus of Religious Studies and Director of the Centre for the Cross-Cultural Study of Health and Healing, Department of Family Medicine, University of Alberta. Dr. Waugh focused his early research and writing on two cultural areas critical today—Islamic studies and Indigenous studies. He has written or edited over a dozen books, dictionaries, and studies, and has received several awards for his writings. Dr. Waugh lectures and consults widely on health care and culture and has provided seminars for health professionals. In 2005, he received the prestigious Salvos Prelorentzos Award for Peace Education by Project Ploughshares for his commitment to education about minority groups. The Alberta College of Pharmacists and the Alberta Pharmacists' Association honoured him with a Friend of Pharmacy award in 2010.

Kyle Y.T. Whitfield completed her PHD at the University of Waterloo in the School of Planning, Ontario, Canada. Her work as a community planner for a mainly rural-based specialized geriatric service in 1995 sparked her inspiration to continue to further enhance health services in rural communities in Canada. She is passionate about exploring the use of models and approaches that are more inclusive of vulnerable people in the decision-making process about health services. Her background in community development and community-based research, rural extension studies, health service planning, aging, and palliative and end-of-life care continues to add to knowledge through her research, community service, and teaching.

Allison Williams completed her PHD at York University, Toronto, Canada, and after holding positions at both Brock University and University of Saskatchewan, is now an Associate Professor in McMaster University's School of Geography and Earth Sciences. Her background in social and health geography continue to contribute to interdisciplinary research teams, three of which are examining urban quality of life, informal palliative caregiving, and rural health service delivery.

Donna M. Wilson is a Registered Nurse, with a full-time tenured or continuing position as a Professor in the Faculty of Nursing, University of Alberta. In 2005, she was offered and accepted a joint-appointment as Caritas Nurse Scientist. Caritas is a faith-based organization that operates two of Edmonton's major acute-care hospitals and a multipurpose continuing-care facility. She also works part time as a casual staff nurse in a local acute-care hospital to remain current in health care and nursing practice. Dr. Wilson's education includes a three-year diploma in nursing from the Royal Alexandra Hospital School in Edmonton (1976), a Baccalaureate in Nursing degree (University of Alberta, 1981), a Master of Science in Nursing degree (University of Texas at Austin, 1985), and a Doctor of Philosophy in Educational Administration degree (University of Alberta, 1993). She has worked in Alberta, British Columbia, New Zealand, and Texas as a staff nurse, nursing supervisor, hospital administrator, nurse educator, and health researcher. Dr. Wilson's program of research focuses on health services utilization and health policy, primarily in relation to aging and end-of-life care. Her research often involves large administrative or population databases and mixed-methods to incorporate both qualitative and quantitative data.

David Young spent his childhood in Sierra Leone. After receiving his PHD from Stanford University in 1970, he taught anthropology at the University of Alberta until 1999 when he accepted a teaching position in Japan. Dr. Young has conducted fieldwork in Mexico, Japan, China, and Alberta. A primary interest has been the healing practices of indigenous peoples. He is retired and living on Vancouver Island.

INDEX

malaria, 100–01
medical culture
  in China, 115
  and ethical behaviour, 82–84
  explanation of, 80–82
  and language, 157–59
  and L-CAP, 168
medical education programs,
  78–80, 84–87
menopause
  biomedical view of, 210–14,
    220–21, 222
  ethnic experience of, 206,
    216–20, 221–22
  socio-cultural view of, 214–15
meta-models, 253–54, 256, 257
Moostoos (medicine man), 249, 250
multiculturalism, xi–xii
Multiple Mini Interview, 94–95
Muslims, 23, 26, 27, 28, 29, 30, 179

Objective Structured Clinical Exam
  (OSCE)
  described, 92–93
  and L-CAP, 167, 168–69
  as major IMG hurdle, 137
  scores of applicants from India
    and China, 122–23
  as test of language proficiency,
    152–53, 159
observerships, 136, 137, 139, 168–69

Pakistan, 112, 113, 114, 116, 117, 140
palliative care
  and Aboriginal peoples, 6–7,
    9–12, 13–15
  change agents for in Alberta,
    44–45, 51, 57
  community based, 36–37
  government commitment to,
    50–51, 52, 53–54
  and home care, 48–49
  key informants' questionnaire
    on, 61–63
  key informants' view of, 43–44
  and long-term care needs,
    49–50
  and reduction of regional
    health authorities, 45–46, 58

  in rural areas, 46–47, 48, 49, 54, 55–56
  successful programs of, 54–56, 58–59
  suggestions for future, 13–15, 56–57
  timeline of Alberta policy on, 39–42
  traditional methods of, xvi
Pallium Project, 36, 47, 58
personal autonomy, 8–9
personal directives, 29
physician preceptors, 95, 97
primary care, 52–53, 56
psoriasis, 249, 251
public education, 185

racism, 193, 194
rattle ceremony, 250–51
recency effect, 155–56
residency training, 71–73, 98–99, 134–35,
  141, 168
resuscitation, 29–30
Rose (medicine man helper), 263, 266, 267
rural areas
  and consultation with urban areas, 50
  problems of palliative care in, 46–47,
    48, 49
  and successful palliative care, 54,
    55–56

seniors
  demographics of, 228, 243
  as part of health services study, 232–39
  and use of health services, 227–29,
    231–32, 234, 235–36, 238, 244, 246
shaking tipi ceremony, 250
Simulated Office Oral (SOO) exam, 73
Somali-Canadians, 219–20
spatial inequality, 120
spontaneous healing, 249, 251, 256–58

telehealth, 54
Thomas, T.G., 211
Tilt, Edward, 210–11
traditional medicines, 8
translators. See interpreters/translators

visa doctors, 152
visible minorities
  demographics of, 228, 243, 245
  and healthy immigrant effect, 236–37
  as part of health services study, 232–39

FIGURE 1: *Country of Medical School Education for All Applicants*

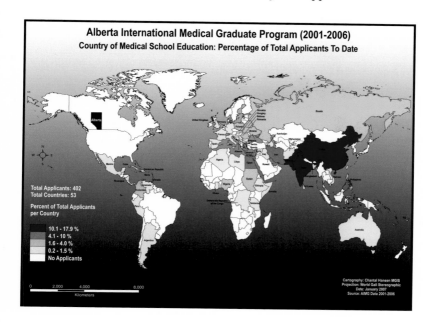

FIGURE 2: *Country of Medical School Education for Successful Applicants*

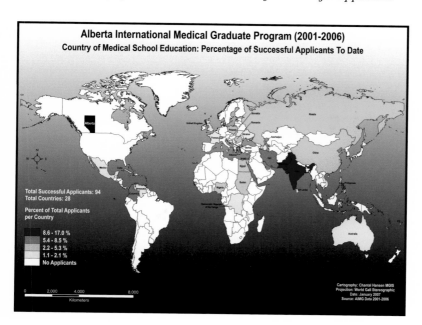

FIGURE 3: *Applicant Country of Medical Education:*
Primary Language of Instruction

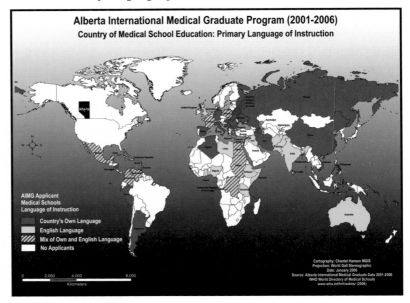

FIGURE 4: *Applicant Country of Medical Education:*
Gender Dominance Among Applicants

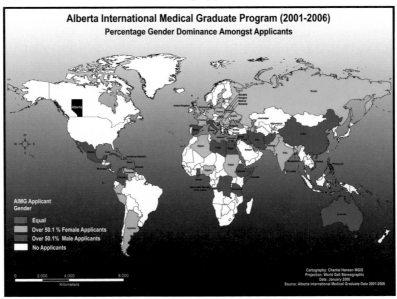

FIGURE 5: *Country of Medical School Education for 2001 Applicants*

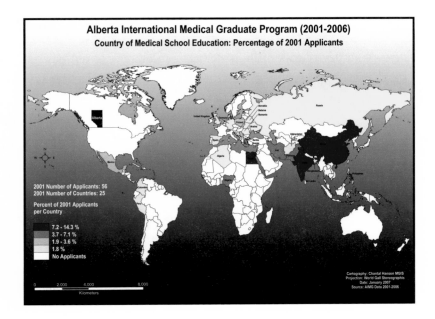

FIGURE 6: *Country of Medical School Education for 2006 Applicants*

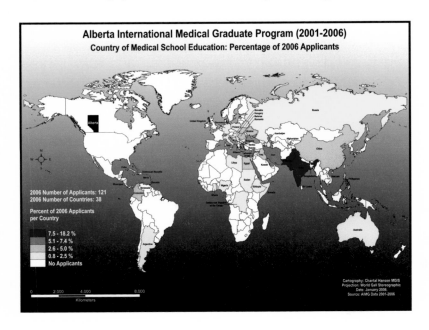

FIGURE 7: *Immigration to Alberta 2004*

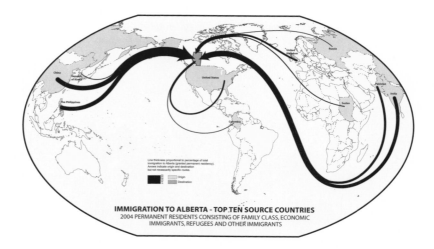

IMMIGRATION TO ALBERTA - TOP TEN SOURCE COUNTRIES
2004 PERMANENT RESIDENTS CONSISTING OF FAMILY CLASS, ECONOMIC
IMMIGRANTS, REFUGEES AND OTHER IMMIGRANTS